Anabolic Steroids and Sports and Drug Testing: 1991-1997

Anabolic Steroids and Sports and Drug Testing: 1991-1997

An Annotated Bibliography

Compiled by
Ellen R. Paterson

The Whitston Publishing Company
Troy, New York
1998

Libraray of Congress Catalog Card Number 97-62104

ISBN 0-87875-499-7

Printed in the United States of America

Contents

Preface

This publication is an updated and expanded continuation of my earlier book-bibliography, *Anabolic Steroids and Sports*, published in 1991. Many more articles have been published in the area of drug testing of college and high school and even elementary school athletes after the controversial Supreme Court majority decision in Vernonia School District 47J v. Acton of 1995. There are numerous well-written and thoroughly reviewed legal discussions of privacy and the Fourth and Fourteenth Amendments to the U.S. Constitution, court cases from lower courts explained and analyzed, and the legal defense explored involving the use of anabolic steroids and violent behavior. The NCAA, several large university, and the Vernonia School District's drug testing policies and procedures are compared. The Anabolic Steroids Control Act of 1990, federal and state constitutional limitations and search and seizure issues are examined. There are articles on the psychological and physical effects or changes associated with anabolic steroid use as well as new books and articles on the potential anti-aging effects of superhormone supplements, such as: DHEA and melatonin. There are sections on children and adolescents along with drug education and prevention efforts and use surveys which mostly sampled high school or college students. The emphasis for this update was on longer review articles and thus shorter newspaper and popular magazine articles are rarely cited and briefly annotated. As in the previous edition, articles that were exclusively reports of animal studies are omitted along with foreign language articles other than English. There are well over five hundred and fifty references to books, chapters, videos, theses, pamphlets, and periodical articles cited and annotated and these cover the years 1991 through the summer of 1997, with some older articles that were missed in the first edition. I made very thorough use of table of contents current awareness alerting services, namely CARL UnCover and FirstSearch's ArticleFirst, full-text periodical databases, and traditional indexes and abstracts. A glossary has once again been provided with medical, legal and slang terms or expressions frequently encountered. First and second authors are cited, first authors indexed, and a brief subject index provided.

Ellen R. Paterson
10/9/97

List of Journals Cited

ABA Journal
Academe
Acta Endocrinologica
Acta Psychiatrica Scandinavia
Addiction and Recovery
Addictive Behaviors
Adelaide Law Review
Adolescence
Adolescent Medicine
Advances in Internal Medicine
Advances in Pediatrics
Aggressive Behavior
AIDS and Public Policy Journal
Albany Law Review
AMA Guidelines for Adolescent Preventive Services
American Criminal Law Review
American Entomologist
American Family Physician
American Health
American Heart Journal
American Journal of Addictions
American Journal of the Diseases of Children
American Journal of Drug and Alcohol Abuse
American Journal of Emergency Medicine
American Journal of Gastroenterology
American Journal of the Medical Sciences
American Journal of Obstetrics and Gynecology
American Journal of Psychiatry
American Journal of Sports Medicine
American Journal on Addictions
American Pharmacy
American Secondary Education
Analytical Chemistry
Annals of Clinical Psychiatry
Annals of Internal Medicine
Annals of Pharmacotherapy
Applied Research in Coaching and Athletics Annual (ARCAA)
Archives of Family Medicine
Archives of General Psychiatry
Archives of Gerontology and Geriatrics
Archives of Internal Medicine
Archives of Pediatrics and Adolescent Medicine
Archives of Sexual Behavior
Arizona State Law Journal
Arkansas Law Review

Athletic Business
Australian Journal of Public Administration
Aviation, Space, and Environmental Medicine
Better Nutrition for Today's Living
Biological Mass Spectrometry
Biological Psychiatry
Biotechnology
Bone and Mineral
British Journal of Sports Medicine
British Medical Journal
Brooklyn Law Review
Buffalo Physician and Biomedical Scientist
Bulletin on Narcotics
Business Week
Canadian Journal of Psychiatry
Canadian Medical Association Journal
Cardiology
Catholic University Law Review
Cato Journal
Chemical and Engineering News
Chemistry and Industry
China Quarterly
Chiropractic Sports Medicine
Clinical Chemistry
Clinical Journal of Sport Medicine
Clinical Pediatrics
Clinical Pharmacy
Clinical Science
Coach and Athletic Director
Comprehensive Psychiatry
Comprehensive Therapy
CQ Researcher
Creighton Law Review
Current Health 2
Cutis
Denver University Law Review
Diagnosis
Dickinson Law Review
Drug and Alcohol Dependence
Drugs in Sports
Education Digest
Education Law Reporter
Endocrine Reviews
Endocrinology and Metabolism Clinics of North America
Far Eastern Economic Review
FASEB Journal
FBI Law Enforcement Bulletin
FDA Consumer
Fitness and Sports Review International
Harvard Journal of Law and Public Policy
Hastings International and Comparative Law Review
Healthy Weight Journal
Hofstra Law Review
Hormones and Behavior
Houston Law Review
Howard Law Journal
Human Psychopharmacology
ICHPER-SP Journal

Medical Clinics of North America
Medicine and Science in Sports and Exercise
Men's Health
Michigan Law Review
Military Law Review
Military Medicine
Minnesota Law Review
Modern Medicine of Australia
Muscular Development
NASSP Bulletin
National Institute on Drug Abuse Research Monograph Series
National Law Journal
National Strength and Conditioning Association Journal
Nebraska Law Review
New England Journal of Medicine
New Jersey Medicine
New Law Journal
New Scientist
New Statesman and Society
New York Law School Journal of Human Rights
Newsweek
North Carolina Law Review
North Dakota Law Review
Nutrition Forum
Nutrition Today
Oregon Law Review
Orthopedic Clinics of North America
Ottawa Law Review
Palaestra
Parade Magazine
Pediatric Exercise Science
Pediatrics
Perceptual and Motor Skills
Pharmaceutical Journal
Pharmacological Research
Phi Delta Kappan
Physical Educator
Physical Medicine and Rehabilitation Clinics of North America
Physical Therapy
Physician and Sports Medicine
Postgraduate Medicine
Prevention Pipeline
Primary Cardiology
Psychiatric Annals
Psychoneuroendocrinology
Obesity Research
Quarterly Journal of Ideology
Research Quarterly for Exercise and Sport
Running Times
Rutgers Law Review
Saint Louis University Law Journal
Scholastic Coach
School Business Affairs
School Law Bulletin
Science
Science News
Sciences
Scientific American

Search
Self
Seton Hall Journal of Sport Law
Seton Hall Law School Constitutional Law Journal
Skin Diver
South African Medical Journal
South Texas Law Review
Southern California Law Review
Southern Medical Journal
Sport Health
Sport Psychologist
Sports and the Courts
Sports Illustrated
Sports Law: Cases and Materials
Sports Lawyers Journal
Sports Medicine
Sports Medicine Digest
Sports Medicine, Training and Rehabilitation
Stanford Journal of International Law
Strength and Conditioning
Suffolk University Law Review
Swimming World and Junior Swimmer
Texas Monthly
Texas Tech Law Review
Therapeutic Drug Monitoring
Thomas M. Cooley Law Review
Thrombosis and Haemostasis
Time
Tips for Principals
Track Technique
Trends in Pharmacological Sciences
Trial
Tulsa Law Journal
Ultrafit
University of Chicago Legal Forum
University of Colorado Law Review
University of Hawaii Law Review
University of Kansas Law Review
University of Miami Entertainment and Sports Law Review
University of Michigan Journal of Law Reform
University of San Francisco Law Review
University of Toledo Law Review
US News and World Report
Valparaiso University Law Review
Washington Law Review
Wayne Law Review
West Virginia Law Review
Western Journal of Medicine
Whittier Law Review
Widener Journal of Public Law
William and Mary Law Review
Wilson Quarterly
Wisconsin Law Review
Women's Sports and Fitness

Books, Films, Videos, Theses, Pamphlets

ANABOLIC STEROIDS: QUEST FOR SUPERMAN. Human Relations Media, 1992. 30 minutes. Pleasantville, New York.
  Reviews medical and nonmedical use, emphasizes problems, interviews users, and presents an anti-steroid message.

ANABOLIC STEROIDS: ROID ROULETTE: A DANGEROUS GAME. Toledo: Media Production Group, 1991. 42 minutes.
  A football coach is the host for this video on steroid use by athletes with suggestions for intervention by parents and coaches.

Anshel, M. H. "Psychology of drug use," Chapter 40, pp. 851-876, in HANDBOOK OF RESEARCH ON SPORT PSYCHOLOGY. New York: MacMillan, 1993.
  Extremely thorough review of the psychological reasons for drug use in sport as well as social causes. Possible intervention strategies are also reviewed.

Bahrke, M. S. and C. E. Yesalis. "Psychological/behavioral effects of anabolic-androgenic steroids," Chapter 41, pp. 877-887, in HANDBOOK OF RESEARCH ON SPORT PSYCHOLOGY. New York: McMillan, 1993.
  Thorough discussion of androgen therapy and the treatment of mental disorders and AAS dependence. Authors suggest that mental health has improved through anabolic steroid use, but recommend further studies; extensive references.

Bellino, F. L., et al. DEHYDROEPIANDROSTERONE (DHEA) AND AGING. Washington, D.C.: New York Academy of Sciences, June 17-19, 1995, Volume 774.
  This is a collection of research papers gathered as a result of a conference. It includes overviews and research challenges, technical reports and studies on biosynthesis of DHEA, physiology, immunology, etc.

BENNY AND THE 'ROIDS. Walt Disney Educational Media, Coronet/MTI Film & Video, 1988. 22 minutes.
  Dangers are dramatized using the character Benny Zimmer, linebacker for high school team, who purchases AAS and gets side effects. Message is that hard work and good health are real winners.

Bhasin, S., et al. BIOLOGY, PHARMACOLOGY, AND CLINICAL APPLICATIONS OF ANDROGENS: CURRENT STATUS AND FUTURE PROSPECTS. International Androgen Workshop, 2nd, 1995, Long Beach, California. Wiley-Liss, 1996.
  Includes chapters on androgen abuse by athletes, testosterone and aggression, and androgen therapy.

Brower, K. J. "Anabolic-Androgenic Steroids," in COMPREHENSIVE HAND-
BOOK OF DRUG AND ALCOHOL ADDICTION, edited by N. S. Miller.
Dekker, 1991, pp. 521-536.
Excellent overview on AAS: history, pharmacology, epidemiology, patterns of use, medical and psychiatric effects, dependence, identification
and assessment, treatment, detoxification, rehabilitation, prevention and
references.

—. "Anabolic Steroids," in the ENCYCLOPEDIA OF DRUGS AND ALCOHOL,
Volume 1, MacMillan, 1995. pp. 117-122.
This provides a good overview on AASs with definitions, controlled
status, chemical structure, generic and brand names, uses, potential side
effects, addictive potential, and more.

Bucci, L. NUTRITION APPLIED TO INJURY REHABILITATION AND SPORTS
MEDICINE. Boca Raton: CRC Press, 1995.
Covers dietary guidelines, proteins, amino acids, vitamins and minerals,
etc.

—. NUTRIENTS AS ERGOGENIC AIDS FOR SPORT AND EXERCISE. Boca
Raton: CRC, 1993.
Covers supplements, macronutrients, amino acids, minerals, etc.

BULKING UP: THE DANGERS OF STEROIDS. Van Nuys, California: AIMS
Media, 1990. 23 minutes.
Bruce Jenner hosts, describing the harmful effects.

Cherniske, S. THE DHEA BREAKTHROUGH. New York: Ballentine, 1996.
This biochemist and sports nutritionist enthusiastically promotes exercise,
stress management, dietary changes, and DHEA along with other supplements; he does not support taking supplements without proper testing and
medical supervision and warns that melatonin has become a fad and is
misused by many. Author explains studies that have shown that DHEA has
anticancer and cardioprotective properties. He also makes some comparisons with testosterone, growth hormone, etc.; extensive references.

Clark, N. NANCY CLARK'S SPORTS NUTRITION GUIDEBOOK. 2nd ed.
Champaign, Illinois: Human Kinetics, 1997.
Includes chapters on protein training and energy-rich foods that build
muscle and nutrition before and during exercise to peak performance,
and more.

Clayton, L. STEROIDS. New York: Rosen, 1996.
This is a very simple, basic introduction for children and young adults. It
has black and white and color photographs, charts, case studies, glossary, index, further reading, etc. It covers history, types of steroids, how
they work, side effects, and people who can help; promotes drug-free
choice as part of drug abuse prevention library.

Courson, S. and L. R. Schreiber. FALSE GLORY: STEELERS AND STEROIDS:
THE STEVE COURSON STORY. Stamford, Connecticut: Longmeadow
Press, 1991.
Details his own drug use of a variety of AAS as well as alcohol starting in
college and escalating as a Pittsburgh Steeler and continuing after brief
time with Tampa Bay. Also comments on drug use in professional football,
coaches looking the other way, less than serious response of the NFL, etc.
No index but very readable and informative. Courson maintains that
negative effects have been exaggerated despite his rare heart problem.

Day, R. B. LEGAL ISSUES SURROUNDING SAFE SCHOOLS. Topeka, Kansas: National Organization on Legal Problems of Education (NOLPE), 1994.
> Chapter V, "Search and Seizure," pp. 25-38, includes discussion of the Fourth Amendment, selected cases, urinalysis testing, metal detector and canine searches.

Dise, J. H., Jr., et al. SEARCHES OF STUDENTS, LOCKERS AND AUTOMOBILES. Detroit, Michigan: Educational Risk, 2d. ed., 1996.
> Section 3.1.2 (pp. 39-44) is devoted to drug testing and a review of selected appropriate cases (Schaill v. Tippecanoe, T.L.O., Vernonia, etc.). Authors warn school districts to check with their attorneys regarding individual state constitutions before implementing any drug testing. Other proposals since Vernonia are briefly reported.

DRUG USE AND SPORT: CURRENT ISSUES AND IMPLICATIONS FOR PUBLIC HEALTH. Geneva: WHO, 1993.
> Overview from an international perspective including the role of WHO, different drugs, efforts to control, etc.

Duchaine, D. UNDERGROUND STEROID HANDBOOK II. Marina Del Ray, California: Power Distributors, Update 1992.
> Underground steroid handbook for men and women includes clenbuterol, cytaden as well as anabolic steroids.

Elster, A. B. and N. J. Kuznets. "Rationale and recommendations: use of alcohol, other drugs, and anabolic steroids," in AMA GUIDELINES FOR ADOLESCENT PREVENTIVE SERVICES, Chapter 11, pp. 117-129. Chicago: American Medical Association, Department of Adolescent Health, 1994.
> Excellent overview of use, consequences, how to identify users, intervention, and extensive references cited.

Fahey, T. STEROID ALTERNATIVE HANDBOOK. Understanding Anabolic Steroids and Drug-Free Scientific Natural Alternatives. San Jose, California: Sport Science Publications, April 1991.
> About one-third of this guide is devoted to basic, simple review, definitions, explanations and the rest to alternatives such as: cycle training, mind/ vision, diet; extensive references but no index.

Francis, C. and J. Coplon. SPEED TRAP: INSIDE THE BIGGEST SCANDAL IN OLYMPIC HISTORY. New York: St. Martin, 1990.
> Sprinter Ben Johnson's track coach presents his side of the international track scene, insisting that chemical assistance should be a personal choice and that health hazards of AAS are greatly exaggerated.

Fuentes, R. J. and J. M. Rosenberg. ATHLETIC DRUG REFERENCE '94. Durham, North Carolina: Clean Data, 1994.
> Fuentes and Rosenberg are authors of chapter 2, "Anabolic Steroids and the Athlete," as well as editors of the handbook which complies with NCAA and USOC rules. Chapter 3 covers drug testing procedures for the athlete. Editors provide very readable descriptions, medical uses, adverse effects, use by athletes, legal issues, etc.; many references cited.

Goldman, B. and R. Klatz. DEATH IN THE LOCKER ROOM: DRUGS AND SPORTS. Chicago, Illinois: Elite Sports Medicine, 1992, 2nd ed.
> Revised edition of 1984 publication which has vital information on women and AAS, growth hormone, drugs and sports and society, drug detection, nutritional ergogenics, sport psychology, and much more.

3

Green, T. "Creating the Perfect Beast: Steroids, Amphetamines and Human Growth Hormones," pp. 76-81, in DARK SIDE OF THE GAME: MY LIFE IN THE NFL. New York: Warner, 1996.
  Brief essay and commentary from Syracuse University's famous alumnus.

Holstein, M. "Sports and Drugs," Chapter 9, pp. 239-263, in UPPERS, DOWNERS, ALL AROUNDERS: PHYSICAL AND MENTAL EFFECTS OF PSYCHOACTIVE DRUGS. San Francisco: CNS Productions, 2nd ed., 1993.
  Thorough overview including history, advertisements, extent of abuse, different kinds of drugs, side effects, policies, identification and referral; illustrated and readable.

Husch, J. A. DRUG USE AND SPORT: CURRENT ISSUES AND IMPLICATIONS FOR PUBLIC HEALTH. Geneva: WHO, 1993.
  Summarizes global trends, current drug use patterns, international responses, WHO activities, etc.; very thorough overview.

Jackson, C. G. R. NUTRITION FOR THE RECREATIONAL ATHLETE. Boca Raton: CRC, 1995.
  This book includes dietary guidelines, exercise and fitness recommendations, weight loss programs, etc. but only brief information about AAS.

Kalimi, M. and W. Regelson, editors. BIOLOGIC ROLE OF DEHYDROEPIAN-DROSTERONE (DHEA). New York: de Gruyter, 1990.
  Very technical book on the precursor steroid or "buffer hormone."

Karch, S. B. PATHOLOGY OF DRUG ABUSE. New York: CRC, 1996. Chapter 6, "Anabolic Steroids," pp. 409-430.
  This covers pharmacology, clinical indications, steroid-related disorders, abuse, black market, side effects, detecting steroid abuse, profile of a steroid abuser, doping and testing; and extensive references.

Kies, C. V. and J. A. Driskell, editors. SPORTS NUTRITION: MINERALS AND ELECTROLYTES. Boca Raton: CRC, 1995.
  Another in the series on Nutrition and Exercise in Sport, this one covers magnesium, iron, calcium, zinc, carboelectrolyte, etc.

Klein, A. M. LITTLE BIG MEN: BODYBUILDING SUBCULTURE AND GENDER CONSTRUCTION. Albany: SUNY, 1993.
  Book on bodybuilding which includes several discussions of AAS and growth hormone as well as cultural aspects. There is a chapter on women's bodybuilding and the history of the sport from beauty contest to serious competition.

Kochakian, C. D. ANABOLIC-ANDROGENIC STEROIDS. New York: Springer-Verlag, 1976. Ryan, A. J., "Athletics," pp. 515-534 and Addendum VII, pp. 723-725.
  This book reviews related animal research, but also studies on male weightlifters critical of those that found gains with AAS because they were not double-blind and relied on self-reporting and low sample numbers.

Kopera, H. ANABOLIC-ANDROGENIC STEROIDS TOWARDS THE YEAR 2000. Wien: Blackwell-MZV, 1993.
  This book covers the chemistry, pharmacology, clinical uses, side effects, etc. Includes a chapter, "Anabolic Steroids in Athletes," pp. 231-261, written by Yesalis, Wright & Lombardo. Text in English and German.

Kurz, T. SCIENCE OF SPORTS TRAINING: HOW TO PLAN AND CONTROL
TRAINING FOR PEAK PERFORMANCE. Island Pond Vermont: Stadion, 1991.
Brief mention of AAS, but mostly on athletic training for speed, endurance, coordination, agility, flexibility, strength, and psychological
advantage.

Kusserow, R. P. ADOLESCENTS AND STEROIDS. Washington, D.C.: Department of Health and Human Services, 1990. (OEI-06-90-01081).
Describes adolescent steroid use patterns, reasons for use, effects,
awareness of risks, all from 72 former and/or current steroid uses; com-
panion report, ADOLESCENT STEROID USE by Tyler.

Laron, Z. and A. D. Rogol, editors. HORMONES AND SPORT. New York: Raven,
1989.
Papers are gathered from a symposium on acute and possible long term
effects of physical exercise and sport on hormone secretion, physical
growth, puberty, nutrition, etc.; D. R. Lamb has a paper, "Anabolic
Steroids and Athletic Performance," and there are others on strength
training, urinary testosterone, and more.

Lowcock, P. W. ANABOLIC-ANDROGENIC STEROID USE: THE KNOWLEDGE,
ATTITUDES AND BEHAVIOR OF HIGH SCHOOL FOOTBALL PLAYERS.
Thesis. University of Kansas, 1992.
Author includes the AAS portion of the King Drugs in Sport Questionnaire,
1991, and determined that there was a low percentage of uses, many
reported positive effects, and many used for the improvement of appearance. Efficacy of drug education was seriously questioned in terms of
limiting AAS use.

Mellion, M. B., et al. THE TEAM PHYSICIAN'S HANDBOOK. New York: Mosby,
1997.
This book includes chapters on drugs and doping, testing requirements,
drug education, strength training and sports nutrition; extensive references.

Miracle, A. W. LESSONS OF THE LOCKER ROOM. Amherst, New York: Prome-
theus Books, 1994.
AAS are discussed in the chapter briefly under school sport and
delinquency.

Mottram, D. R., editor. DRUGS IN SPORT. New York: Chapman & Hall, 1996.
2nd ed.
Chapters are written by different authors who write about the topics of
drug abuse in sport, different classes of drugs, testing issues, sport injuries and treatment, blood boosting, etc.; glossary and index. "Anabolic
Steroids and Growth Hormone" are discussed in Chapter 7, pp. 173-218.

Munro, R. ANABOLIC STEROIDS: KNOWLEDGE, ATTITUDE, AND BEHAVIOR
IN COLLEGE AGE STUDENTS. Arizona State University, 1991.
This thesis includes information on weight training and sport psychology
as well as AAS.

Myers, M. COMPULSIVE EXERCISE AND STEROID ABUSE. Park Ridge, Illinois:
Parkside Publishing Corporation, 1990, 32 p.
This is a pamphlet size overview of the history/reasons/side effects/
methods/dangers/withdrawal/HGH/brief personal testimonies, etc.

Park & Park, et al. "Mass Spectrometry in Sports Testing," in FORENSIC APPLI-
CATIONS OF MASS SPECTROMETRY, edited by J. Yinon. Ann Arbor,
Michigan: CRC Press, 1995.
    Brief historical background provided and then very technical and very
    specific screening procedures and analysis along with graphs, charts and
    structures.

Pierpaoli, W. and W. Regelson. THE MELATONIN MIRACLE: NATURE'S AGE-
REVERSING, DISEASE-FIGHTING, SEX-ENHANCING HORMONE. New
York: Simon & Schuster, 1995.
    Authors explain the largely animal research studies that hold such
    promise for melatonin as an anti-cancer and heart protector, but also a
    stress reliever and sleep enhancer, etc. Authors also make recommen-
    dations concerning dosages as well as lifestyle changes.

Regelson, W. and C. Colman. THE SUPERHORMONE PROMISE: NATURE'S
ANTIDOTE TO AGING. New York: Simon and Schuster, 1996.
    This book covers much more than DHEA, but also testosterone, estro-
    gen, progesterone, melatonin, pregnenolone, growth and thyroid hor-
    mone. Authors call the mix the superhormone cocktail and explain well
    the research that has been done concerning DHEA and other supple-
    ments. Regelson co-authored THE MELATONIN MIRACLE.

Ringhofer, K. R. and M. E. Harding. COACHES GUIDE TO DRUGS AND SPORT.
Champaign, Illinois: Human Kinetics, 1996.
    Provides information about AAS and drug testing as well as educational
    resources and other materials for parents and coaches and school staff.

Rogozkin, V. A. METABOLISM OF ANABOLIC ANDROGENIC STEROIDS. Boca
Raton: CRC, 1991.

Rossow, L. F. and J. A. Stefkovich. SEARCH AND SEIZURE IN THE PUBLIC
SCHOOLS. Topeka, Kansas: National Organization of Legal Problems of
Education (NOLPE), 2d. ed., 1995.
    Chapter V, "Searches for Drugs and Drug Testing," pp. 59-68, is a review
    of specific cases regarding privacy, reasonableness standard, drug
    testing of students, including athletes, and individualized suspicion.
    Acton v. Vernonia case is summarized on pp. 63-66.

Scott, R. F. PREVALENCE OF ILLICIT ANABOLIC STEROID USE AMONG
RURAL-AGRARIAN COLLEGE AGE STUDENTS. Sam Houston State
University, 1993. Thesis.
    Discusses rural trends and develops a typology of the rural-agrarian
    college age steroid user; glossary in appendix.

STEROID ALERT. Barr Films, Irwindale, California, 1990. 23 minutes.
    Explains the history of steroid use, how chemical composition affects the
    human body, side effects, and interviews with ex-users.

STEROID TRAP: TURNING WINNERS INTO LOSERS. Guidance Associates, Mt.
Kisco, New York, 1990. 37 minutes. Two videocassettes.
    Explores who uses and why, illustrates side effects, and discusses peer
    pressure.

STEROIDS: THE REAL STORY. Pleasantville, New York: Sunburst, 1993. 27
minutes.
    Four ex-users, two ex-dealers, and one current dealer describe their ex-
    periences, especially with side effects.

STEROIDS: A RESOURCE GUIDE. Albany, New York: University of the State of New York, State Education Department, Division of Pupil Health & Fitness, Bureau of School Health Education & Services, 1991.
>This is a curriculum guide for the study and teaching of AAS abuse.

STEROIDS: STRAIGHT TALK ABOUT STRONG MEDICINE. Northfield, Minnesota: Life Skills Education, 1995.
>Very readable overview, what steroids are, how they work, prevention and education strategies with teachers and coaches in mind.

Stilger, V. G. INDIANA HIGH SCHOOL FOOTBALL PLAYERS' ATTITUDE, KNOWLEDGE, AND USE OF ANABOLIC ANDROGENIC STEROIDS. Thesis. Indiana University, 1993.

Taylor, W. N. MACHO MEDICINE: A HISTORY OF THE ANABOLIC STEROID EPIDEMIC. North Carolina: McFarland & Company, 1991.
>Provides historical background on the discovery and synthesis of testosterone to the reclassification of AAS as narcotics under the Steroid Trafficking Act of 1990. Much of the book is devoted to federal legislation and regulation.

Tricker, R. and D. L. Cook. ATHLETES AT RISK: DRUGS AND SPORT. Dubuque: Brown/Benchmark, 1993.
>Different authors cover such topics as history of sport, ethical issues, AAS, psychological factors, drug testing, etc.

Tyler, J. V., et al. ADOLESCENT STEROID USE. Washington, D.C.: Department of Health and Human Services, 1991. (OEI 06-90-01080).
>Companion report to ADOLESCENTS AND STEROIDS: A USER PERSPECTIVE (OEI-06-90-01081), by Kusserow, that gives comparisons of findings, NIDA statistics, literature review, and more detail.

Van de Loo, D. A. and M. D. Johnson. "Anabolic Steroid Use in Adolescent Athletes," Chapter 14, pp. 226-227, in CHILDREN AND YOUTH IN SPORT, edited by F. I. Smoll and R. E. Smith. McGraw-Hill, 1996.
>Very good overview of the physiological and potential adverse effects, how and why adolescents use, and how to identify and maybe prevent steroid use; extensive references.

Volpert, T. R. and D. W. Tremaine. "Drug Testing of Interscholastic Athletes in Public Schools," 4-1 to 4-7, in the LEGAL HANDBOOK ON SCHOOL ATHLETICS, Alexandria, National School Boards Association, 1997.
>This is a very readable and understandable review of the Vernonia v. Acton Supreme Court case as it directly applies to public school districts. Authors suggest guidelines for establishing drug testing programs based on the Vernonia policy and cite one post-Vernonia case.

Yasser, R. L., J. R. McCurdy and C. P. Goplerud. SPORTS LAW: CASES AND MATERIALS, 3rd ed. Cincinnati: Anderson Publishing Company, 1997.
>Chapter 12, "Drug Testing," pp. 789-822, has a reprint of the Vernonia v. Acton Supreme Court decision (115 S. Ct. 2386 1985) dealing with the testing of junior and senior high public school athletes, followed with a problem designed to address unanswered questions, i.e., "you are a law clerk to the Oklanois state court judge . . .", and "notes and comments" that provides a review, legal references, points for schools, draft guidelines, policy considerations, etc. that distinguish between performance-enhancing substances and recreational drugs.

Yesalis, C. E. ANABOLIC STEROIDS IN SPORT AND EXERCISE. Champaign, Illinois: Human Kinetics, 1993.
This is a collection of fourteen articles organized into three parts: History and Incidence of Use, Effects, Dependence and Treatment, and Testing and Societal Alternatives.

— and M. S. Bahrke. "Psychological/behavioral effects of anabolic-androgenic steroids," Chapter 41, pp. 877-887, in HANDBOOK OF RESEARCH ON SPORT PSYCHOLOGY. New York: McMillan, 1993.
Thorough discussion of androgen therapy and the treatment of mental disorders and AAS dependence. Authors suggest that mental health has improved through anabolic steroid use, but recommend further studies; extensive references.

Zeese, K. B. "Urine Testing of School Students," pp. 8-1 to 8-23, Vol. 2, Chapter 8, in DRUG TESTING. LEGAL MANUAL AND PRACTICE AIDS. Rochester, New York: Clark Boardman Callaghan, 1996, 1997.
This is a very important updated section on testing of high school and college students, including a subsection on steroid testing. Specific cases are cited and reviewed and terms defined and explained along with the Fourth Amendment, NCAA testing program, due process and equal protection requirements, confidentiality, etc. Looseleaf format allows for updating of sections as new legislation is enacted or new cases are decided.

Zemper, E. D. "Drug Testing in Athletics," Chapter 6, pp. 113-139, in DRUG TESTING: ISSUES AND OPTIONS. New York: Oxford University Press, 1991.
Author provides a brief history of drug testing in athletics, problem of anabolic steroids (pp. 123-128), professional, college, high school, amateur, including national and international, drug testing, substances and methods banned by the I.O.C.

Periodical Literature

Overview

This section has review articles that provide very good to excellent overall information regarding the history, chemistry, physiology, side effects, definitions, prevalence of use, research studies, legal and ethical issues, testing, safety, etc. on anabolic-androgenic steroids and other ergogenic drugs and aids. Most have many references for further study.

Anabolic-androgenic steroids: current issues, by C. E. Yesalis and Bahrke. SPORTS MEDICINE 19(5):326-340, 1995.
Excellent overview with balanced perspective on incidence of serious side effects, polypharmacy, use studies; 109 references.

Anabolic steroid abuse, by G. L. Landry and W. A. Primos. ADVANCES IN PEDIATRICS 37:185-205, 1990.
Overview—methods of detection and advice—over 100 references.

Anabolic steroid use to enhance athletes' performance, by G. D. Braunstein. SOUTHERN CALIFORNIA LAW REVIEW 65:373-381, 1991.
Very good overview that reviews androgenic vs. anabolic effects, prevalence of misuse, effectiveness, safety, and adverse effects.

Anabolic steroids: addictive, psychiatric, and medical consequences, by K. J. Brower. AMERICAN JOURNAL ON ADDICTIONS 1(2):100-114, Spring 1992.
This is a comprehensive overview which covers the addiction potential of AAS, mechanism of dependence, psychiatric effects, physical side effects, identification and assessment, and directions for future research, well referenced with 123 citations.

Anabolic steroids and ergogenic aids, by D. O. Hough. AMERICAN FAMILY PHYSICIAN 41:1157-1164, 1990; discussion 43:781, 1991.
Overview article covering history, physiologic effects, other ergogenic aids such as HGH, and extensive lists of references.

Anabolic steroids and growth hormone, by H. A. Haupt. AMERICAN JOURNAL OF SPORTS MEDICINE 21:468-474, 1993.
Excellent updated review of the literature—definitions, effects, legislation; 76 references.

Anabolic steroids: effects as an ergogenic aid for athletes, by J. E. Kotecki. ICHPER-SP JOURNAL 31:11-17, 1994.
> This is an excellent overview article which defines terms, reviews use studies, summarizes effects, research, reasons for use.

Anabolic steroids in the training and treatment of athletes, by T. J. Limbird. COMPREHENSIVE THERAPY 11:25-30, 1985.
> Excellent overview article with definitions which reviews the pharmacology, describes conflicting evidence relating to ergogenic effects, and potential side effects.

Androgen abuse by athletes, by J. D. Wilson. ENDOCRINE REVIEWS 9:181-199, 1988.
> Overview of technical pharmacology, pattern of abuse, side effects; 216 references.

Androgens, brain and behavior, by D. R. Rubinow and P. J. Schmidt. AMERICAN JOURNAL OF PSYCHIATRY 153:974-984, 1996.
> Excellent overview article which summarizes the research studies on androgens (including AAS and DHEA) and behavior; anabolic androgenic steroids have direct behavior effects which have been reported to cause mood disorders and to help some and not others in terms of treating depression.

Assessing the threat of anabolic steroids, by R. H. Strauss. PHYSICIAN AND SPORTS MEDICINE 21:37-41, 44, 1993.
> Four medical experts answer questions about AAS: Don Catlin, Jim Wright, Harrison Pope, and Mariah Liggett; patterns of use, federal laws and supply, clenbuterol, testing and athletes' decline in use, physicians' prescriptions, counseling to discourage use and basics about AAS.

Athletes and drugs, by R. L. Worsnop. CQ RESEARCHER 1:515-535, 1991.
> History of drug policies, literature, legal issues, definitions, drug testing, chronology, photographs, federal and state regulations, notes and annotated bibliography.

Chemical warfare: battling steroids in athletics, by J. Thurston. MARQUETTE SPORTS LAW JOURNAL 93:93-148, 1990.
> Thorough overview on the history of steroids, physical effects, why athletes take steroids, definitions, side effects, obtaining steroids, testing procedures, NCAA regulations, NFL random testing, Fourth Amendment, high school drug testing, collegiate, equal protection, privacy, and more.

Chinese women and sport: success, sexuality and suspicion, by J. Riordan and D. Jinxia. CHINA QUARTERLY 145:130-152, 1996.
> This is a very thorough overview of sport in Chinese society and culture and the possible reasons for such female success, including some discussion of the drug issue, but also the discipline of Chinese female athletes. However, Chinese female swimmers in great numbers have been caught mainly using anabolic steroids; also canoeists, cyclists, a discus thrower, hurdler, and weight lifters have tested positive for AAS. Comparisons are made with the former East Germany.

Current perspectives on anabolic-androgenic steroid abuse, by S. E. Lukas. TRENDS IN PHARMACOLOGICAL SCIENCES 14:61-68, 1993.
> Overview in light of AAS being added to the Schedule III Controlled Substances Act and plea for epidemiological studies of health conse-

quences of acute and chronic steroid use, well-designed and controlled
performance change studies, better models and standards to study
abuse liability, determination of psychological and behavioral effects of
acute and long-term use, etc.

Drug use update, by G. I. Wadler. MEDICAL CLINICS OF NORTH AMERICA
78:439-455, 1994.
Specific drugs continuously change, therefore Wadler reviews and up-
dates on (EPO) erythropoietin, clenbuterol/salbutamol, human growth
hormone (hGH) as well as AAS . . . including sharing of needle and syringe and thus the benefit of syringe exchange programs. Excellent
overview for physicians but readable for the general audience or consumer.

Drugs in sports, by P. S. Zurer. CHEMICAL AND ENGINEERING NEWS 62:69-
78, April 30, 1984.
Special report on banned drugs, doping, anabolic steroids, testing,
growth hormone, tranquilizer and stimulants, and more.

Effects of anabolic-androgenic steroid uses in athletes: a coaches' guide, by K.
E. Riem and K. G. Hursey. APPLIED RESEARCH IN COACHING AND
ATHLETICS ANNUAL (ARCAA) pp. 15-43, 1993.
Excellent overview that tries to correct misconceptions, such as all AASs
have similar effects including side effects and duration of action, patterns
of use; defines and explains popular and technical terms, i.e. "pump"
means desired state of muscular congestion and "gynecomastia" means
small firm tender mass of breast tissue as a result of AAS use. Substantial
selected references for further review are provided.

Effects of anabolic-androgenic steroids on muscular strength, by J. D. Elashoff,
et al. ANNALS OF INTERNAL MEDICINE 115:387-393, 1991.
AAS may enhance muscle strength in previously trained athletes but not
untrained.

Ergogenic aids, by L. A. Thein, et al. PHYSICAL THERAPY 75:426-439, 1995.
Comprehensive overview and technical discussion of the variety of different performance-enhancing substances; includes epidemiology,
pharmacology, side effects, drug testing, etc.; extensive references.

Ergogenic aids: a means to citius, altius, fortius, and Olympic gold?, by M. H.
Williams. RESEARCH QUARTERLY FOR EXERCISE AND SPORT 67(3
Suppl.):S58-S64, 1996.
Reviews several ergogenic aids, why athletes use them, discusses ethics
of use, and provides references: specifically covers blood doping and
EPO, caffeine, sodium bicarbonate, creatine, glycerol and cites studies.

Ergogenic aids: what athletes are using—and why, by E. R. Eichner. PHYSICIAN
AND SPORTS MEDICINE 25:70-76+, 1997.
Updated review on AAS, HGH, clenbuterol and other beta$_2$ agonists, caffeine, and creatine as ergogenic substances; good and very readable
overview on the variety of substances used in the past and present to
enhance performance and testing measures for T/E ratio, etc.

Ergogenic drug use and the role of the pharmacist, by K. O. Price. AMERICAN
PHARMACY 31:65-68, 1991.
Very readable overview of history, ethical and legal issues, information
from pharmacists, and the potential consultative role.

History of anabolic steroids and a review of clinical experience with anabolic steroids, by H. Kopera. ACTA ENDOCRINOLOGICA 271(Suppl.): 11-18, 1995.
>Summarizes animal studies, legitimate medical uses, side effects depending on dose and androgenicity, etc.; references.

History of synthetic testosterone, by J. M. Hoberman and E. Yesalis. SCIENTIFIC AMERICAN, February 1995, pp. 76-81.
>This is an excellent review and history of the use of testosterone and synthetic derivatives, anabolic-androgenic steroids, including clinical uses and sports.

Hormonal ergogenic aids, by A. D. Rogol. JOURNAL OF SPORT REHABILITATION 2:128-140, 1993.
>Very technical article about hGH, erythropoetin, clenbuterol, but not AAS; briefly explains physiology and pharmacology, therapeutic uses, adverse effects, and potential for abuse.

Human growth hormone: physiological functions and ergogenic efficacy, by M. H. Stone. STRENGTH AND CONDITIONING 17:72-74, August 1, 1995.
>Reviews the literature studies on the effectiveness of HGH as an ergogenic aid; summarizes that it does not appear to work and there are harmful side effects; many references.

Is there a rational for growth hormone use in sport, by F. Trudeau. CHIROPRACTIC SPORTS MEDICINE 7:105-108, 1993.
>Another review of the current knowledge of growth hormone as an ergogenic aid, the author concludes that HGH is not an aid in the development of muscle strength in adults; suggests resistance training and good nutrition for strength development.

Listening to steroids, by J. Hoberman. WILSON QUARTERLY 19:35-44, 1995.
>Historical and philosophical discussion of drug use in sports or doping and ethical issues, ergogenic aids, testosterone and its synthetic derivatives, HGH, prozac; author predicts that testosterone products will be used increasingly for AIDS patients and elderly and thus change to legitimate status.

Literature review: anabolic-androgenic steroid use by athletes, by M. H. Stone. NATIONAL STRENGTH AND CONDITIONING ASSOCIATION JOURNAL 15:10-28, 1993. Revised from J. E. Wright and W. H. Stone, NSCAJ 7(5), 1985.
>Clenbuterol and other potentially anabolic drugs added . . . physiological basis, chemical structures, review of research, medical uses, side effects; extensive references.

Medical and nonmedical uses of anabolic-androgenic steroids, by The Council on Scientific Affairs. JAMA 264:2923-2927, December 12, 1990.
>Good overview article that reviews the trends in AAS use, epidemiology, source of the drug, adverse reactions, control efforts, professional education activities, AMA's position and recommendations; 66 references.

Nutrition, anabolic steroids, and growth hormone, by J. R. Jardin, et al. PHYSICAL MEDICINE AND REHABILITATION CLINICS OF NORTH AMERICA 7:253-275, 1996.
>Technical and detailed review of structural chemistry, physiology, animal and human studies, therapeutic use; 112 references.

Of muscles and men, by A. M. Klein. SCIENCES 33(6):32-37, November/
December 1993.
> This cover story features an article adapted and excerpted from Klein's
> book, Little Big Men: Bodybuilding Subculture and Gender Construction,
> SUNY Press, 1993, a social and psychological study of bodybuilding.

Performance-enhancing drugs, by N. A. Ghaphery. ORTHOPEDIC CLINICS OF
NORTH AMERICA 26:433-442, 1995.
> Overview article on prevalence, physiology of testosterone/anabolic
> steroids, side effects as well as growth hormone, erythropoetin, and
> more; drug testing; many references cited.

Polypharmacy: anabolic steroids and beyond, by M. G. Di Pasquale. DRUGS IN
SPORTS 1(1):2-3, 1991.
> Brief introduction to the premier issue.

Psychiatric effects of androgenic and anabolic-androgenic steroid abuse in men: a
brief review of the literature, by D. J. Williamson and A. H. Young. JOURNAL
OF PSYCHOPHARMACOLOGY 6(1):20-26, 1992.
> Technical review of case studies and reports and research studies on
> synthetic sex hormones and depression, dependence/addiction, ag-
> gression/violent behavior, etc.; compares past studies which attempt to
> demonstrate beneficial effects with more recent studies which suggest
> harmful effects in terms of mental illness.

A review of anabolic steroids: uses and effects, by M. LaBree. JOURNAL OF
SPORTS MEDICINE AND PHYSICAL FITNESS 31(4):618-626, 1991.
> Well written and very readable review that covers side effects, AAS used,
> doping control, human and animal studies, but somewhat dated in testing
> decisions which have since been decided; 50 references.

Steroid substitutes, by J. Monroe. CURRENT HEALTH 2, April 1996, pp. 13-15.
> Brief overview of steroid alternatives which are also banned from the
> Olympics; several athletes tested positive and were not allowed to com-
> pete in summer 1992. Clenbuterol, gamma hydroxybutyric, human
> growth hormone, erythropoetin and chromium discussed and examples
> of health risks given.

Steroid substitutes: no-win situation for athletes, by K. L. Ropp. FDA CONSUMER
26:8-12, 1992.
> Overview of the potential health effects of steroid substitutes: clenbuterol,
> growth hormone, and EPO.

Steroid use, by M. Brzycki. COACH AND ATHLETIC DIRECTOR 65(9):75-79,
April 1996.
> This is an overview article on AAS use, side effects, legal status, signs
> and symptoms.

Steroid-using athletes: the body's compartment in an epoch of nihilism, by M. J.
LaFountain and J. R. Fuller. QUARTERLY JOURNAL OF IDEOLOGY 14:1-
18, 1990.
> Philosophical essay that attempts to explain the use of anabolic steroids
> despite the fact that steroid use is not condoned; issues of self-image,
> body and spirit, ego, etc.; references.

Steroids: a spreading peril, by S. Rozin. BUSINESS WEEK June 19, 1995, pp. 138-141.

Excellent readable overview and report on AAS side effects, sources for AAS, drug trafficking and law enforcement efforts, costs, and testing issues in high schools.

Use and abuse of anabolic and other drugs for athletic enhancement, by D. H. Catlin and C. K. Hatton. ADVANCES IN INTERNAL MEDICINE 36:399-424, 1991.

Excellent overview article with 105 references.

Why sports matter, by W. Sheed. WILSON QUARTERLY 19:11-25, 1995.

This is a delightful and thought-provoking essay that covers the history of sport and society. Comparisons are made between coaching and teaching, law and cricket in Trinidad, along with racial, cultural, violence, class issues and values. Soccer in Britain, American football, Japanese and American baseball, market value and individualism, and even the increasing participation of women in competitive sport are all discussed and debated.

Children/Adolescents and Education/Prevention

This section gathers articles on recognizing signs and symptoms of AAS use in teens so that teachers, coaches, parents, counselors, and physicians can identify the AAS user. Peer education and substance abuse prevention programs are described, such as: APPLE, ATLAS and TEAMS. Alternative programs are also recommended that emphasize nutrition and strength training without drugs.

Adolescent steroid use, by J. I. Buckley. Mankato, Minnesota, April 1990, 45 pp. (Report presented in Health Science 631 Graduate Seminar, M.S., Mankato State.)
Review of the literature regarding adolescents with definitions, history, physiological effects, possible long-term effects, reasons adolescents use, sources, role of the health educator, analysis, and health education curriculum.

Adolescents and anabolic steroids: a subject review, by the Committee on Sports Medicine and Fitness. PEDIATRICS 99(6):904-908, June 1997.
This is a revision which provides current information for pediatricians on AAS use by young athletes, i.e. definition, background, how used, side effects, use of other drugs, signs that suggest use, etc. This is a good general overview.

Adolescents Training and Learning to Avoid Steroids (ATLAS) prevention program: background and results of a model intervention, by L. Goldberg, et al. ARCHIVES OF PEDIATRICS AND ADOLESCENT MEDICINE 150:713-722, 1996.
Reports preliminary results from the first year of a four-year study to develop and test a school intervention program to prevent AAS use among male high school football players; provides information about nutrition and strength training.

Anabolic steroid and ergogenic drug use by adolescents, by J. D. Foley and M. Schydlower. ADOLESCENT MEDICINE 4:341-352, 1993.
Excellent overview article on use of AAS, history, testing, costs, withdrawal and dependency, treatment, other ergogenics; references.

Anabolic steroid education and adolescents: do scare tactics work?, by L. Goldberg, et al. PEDIATRICS 87:283-286, 1991.
Recommends a balanced approach using peer education rather than emphasizing adverse side effects; alternatives to drug use such as nutrition and strength training are needed.

Anabolic steroid use in the adolescent athlete, by J. A. Potteiger and V. G. Stilger. JOURNAL OF ATHLETIC TRAINING 29:60-64, 1994.
> AAS use in the adolescent can be detected by trainers who are aware of potential physical and psychological changes; team or family physician should be involved to develop a case history, possible testing and treatment.

Athletic Prevention Programming and Leadership Education (APPLE) model: developing substance abuse prevention programs, by S. J. Grossman, et al. JOURNAL OF ATHLETIC TRAINING 28(2):137-141, Summer 1993.
> Authors describe a program for the prevention of alcohol and other drug (AOD) abuse among student-athletes. This program emphasizes student responsibility and initiative and peer referral. Authors also stress the importance of thorough and effective drug education, including federal, state and local laws and regulations.

Changes in body size of elite high school football players: 1963-1989, by M. Q. Wang, et al. PERCEPTUAL AND MOTOR SKILLS 76:379-383, 1993.
> Authors compare the heights and weights of PARADE MAGAZINE's high school All-American Football Teams and found no significant changes in Body Mass Index for 1963-1971, but an increased pattern in 1972-1989; large increases after 1971 raise questions about the use of AAS.

Effect of an anabolic steroid education program on knowledge and attitudes of high school football players, by L. Goldberg, et al. JOURNAL OF ADOLESCENT HEALTH CARE 11:210-214, 1990.
> Questionnaires were used to assess knowledge and attitudes before and after using the American College of Sports Medicine's position statement on the use of AAS in sports; increased awareness of adverse effects, but no differences in attitudes toward use which was low in the particular teams questioned.

Effects of body image on dieting, exercise, and anabolic steroid use in adolescent males, by A. Drewnowski, et al. INTERNATIONAL JOURNAL OF EATING DISORDERS 17:381-386, 1995.
> Results showed that more adolescent males desire to gain weight rather than lose and typically are more satisfied with their body appearance; number of AAS users was very low.

Effects of a multi-dimensional anabolic steroid prevention intervention, by L. Goldberg, et al. JAMA 276:1555-1562, 1996.
> Reports the first year of a four-year study to reduce factors that encourage AAS use. Peers and coaches are an integral part of the ATLAS program, supported by NIDA grant.

Effects of training at a young age: a review of the Training of Young Athletes (TOYA) study, by A. D. G. Baxter-Jones and P. J. Helms. PEDIATRIC EXERCISE SCIENCE 8:310-327, 1996.
> Reviews the longitudinal study of growth and development of British athletes who participated in gymnastics, soccer, swimming and tennis; negative effects of intensive training were outweighed by social, psychological and health benefits of exercise and sport, specifically aerobic power development and muscular strength, etc.

Ensuring the health of the adolescent athlete, by the Council on Scientific Affairs, AMA. ARCHIVES OF FAMILY MEDICINE 2(4):446-448, 1993.
> This report with recommendations adopted as amended also includes statistics about use and reasons for substance abuse by adolescent

athletes . . . AMA concludes that the preparticipation athletic examination (PAE) is an appropriate time to investigate risk behaviors and to provide adolescent health information about hazards of smoking, drug use and sexually transmissible diseases and unwanted pregnancies.

An evaluation of strategies developed to prevent substance abuse among student-athletes, by R. J. Marcello, et al. SPORT PSYCHOLOGIST 3:196-211, 1989.
Evaluates selected prevention programs, including assessment tools, inventories, etc. and future recommendations.

Everything kids should know about performance-enhancing drugs . . . but were afraid to ask, by L. Melina. SWIMMING WORLD AND JUNIOR SWIMMER 37:34-35, 1996.
Briefly gives an overview and warns that over-the-counter preparations and subscription drugs can be banned and that parents, athletes, coaches, physicians, etc. must understand what is currently banned; provides USOC hotline toll-free phone number.

Fortifying students against steroid use, by L. Schnirring. PHYSICIAN AND SPORTS MEDICINE 24:15-16, 1996.
News brief on the preliminary results of the ATLAS program funded through NIDA.

High-risk behaviors in teenage male athletes, by E. S. Forman, et al. CLINICAL JOURNAL OF SPORT MEDICINE 5:36-42, 1995.
Results suggest that athletic participation by male athletes may lead to a significant decrease in drug and alcohol use and abuse.

Intercollegiate sports participation and non-medical drug use, by J. V. Toohey and B. W. Corder. BULLETIN ON NARCOTICS 33:23-27, 1981.
Study to determine if competitive swimming could modify non-medical drug use.

Intervention and prevention of steroid use in adolescents, by D. Elliot and L. Goldberg. AMERICAN JOURNAL OF SPORTS MEDICINE 24:S46-S47, 1996.
Report of a study of high school football players seems to confirm poly-drug use and that higher-intent students need training in refusal skills; authors expect to use information to prioritize curricular items.

Middle school students' attitudes and use of anabolic steroids, by J. Nutter. JOURNAL OF STRENGTH AND CONDITIONING RESEARCH 11:35-39, 1997.
Study demonstrates the importance of health and physical education teachers in providing information about AAS; also revealed the lack of information in that one-third did not know dangerous side effects. Suggests that parents, coaches, etc. need to be proactive.

Preventing teen drug use. CQ RESEARCHER 5:657-680, July 28, 1995.
This whole issue is devoted to the topic of drug use among youth, including high school sports, coaching, drug testing of athletes, and more; thorough overview of the issues.

Sports pharmacy: counseling athletes about banned drugs, by M. A. Goldwire and K. O. Price. AMERICAN PHARMACY NS35:24-30, May 1995.
Good overview with organizations described, definitions, lists of drugs and some suggestions for education. Also compares the NCAA and USOC banned categories. 40 references.

Spotting the young steroid abuser, by J. A. Lombardo. DIAGNOSIS 10:57-62, 1988.
  Describes physical and behavioral changes that may indicate anabolic steroid use, especially sudden weight gain and aggressiveness.

Student steroid abuse, by R. J. Kusma. EDUCATION DIGEST 61:66-68, March 1996, from TIPS FOR PRINCIPALS December 1995, pp. 1-2, NASSP.
  Good general audience introduction to AAS, brief historical background, reasons for use, side effects, jargon, signs to observe and take note, records to keep, especially for physical education teachers and coaches.

Substance abuse prevention program for student-athletes, by P. W. Meilman and R. L. Fleming. JOURNAL OF COLLEGE STUDENT DEVELOPMENT 31: 477-479, 1990.
  Brief description of an approach to alcohol and drug abuse that covers performance enhancing drugs, alcohol, behaviors, problem use, etc.; strong support and involvement of coaches and athletes at Dartmouth.

Taking a strong stance against anabolic steroid use, by L. A. Wilkerson. JOURNAL OF THE AMERICAN OSTEOPATHIC 95:468-470, 1995.
  Editorial provides a quick overview, adverse side effects, and counseling suggestions; steroid-free drug education programs recommended.

T.E.A.M.S. Teaching and educating athletes against the misuse of substances, by L. B. Jackson. AMERICAN SECONDARY EDUCATION 21:15-18, 1992.
  Describes a substance abuse program which prepares student athletes to become educators and mentors for at-risk students in order to keep them in school and drug free.

Use Surveys

This section includes articles on self-reported use, knowledge about anabolic androgenic steroids, observations of coaches and others, perceptions, beliefs, and attitudes about AAS use, etc. mostly concerning high school and college students in the U.S. and Canada. Most compare AAS to cigarette, alcohol, and other drug use. Many users are not participating in school or college athletics, but use AAS to improve their appearance. Participation in sports may deter AAS use. Most stress the importance of drug education for young adolescents.

Adolescent anabolic-androgenic steroid use, multiple drug use, and high school sports participation, by R. H. DuRant, et al. PEDIATRIC EXERCISE SCIENCE 9:150-158, 1997.
    Compares frequency of AAS use and other illicit drug use with participation in school sports based on a sample of students in grades 9-12 in Massachusetts; frequency of strength training weakly correlated with frequency of AAS use and differences were noted between males and females, polydrug use and school sports participation.

Adolescent body image and attitudes to anabolic steroid use, by E. M. Komoroski, et al. AMERICAN JOURNAL OF THE DISEASES OF CHILDREN 146:823-828, 1992.
    Survey results from eleventh grade central Arkansas high school students; adolescent AAS user may start a life-long dependency to augment body image and participate in athletics.

Anabolic-androgenic steroid use among California Community College student-athletes, by R. D. Kersey. JOURNAL OF ATHLETIC TRAINING 31:237-241, 1996.
    Sample of steroid users tended to be older males, more often minorities, who obtained steroids from illegal sources; most used multiple drugs, believed they knew about steroids, but their information was from lifting partners and fellow athletes.

Anabolic-androgenic steroid use by private health club/gym athletes, by R. D. Kersey. JOURNAL OF STRENGTH AND CONDITIONING RESEARCH 7:118-126, 1993.
    Survey of users of five private health clubs/gyms, regarding their strength training habits and methods, knowledge and use of AAS, demographics; questionnaire included.

Anabolic-androgenic steroid use in the United States, by C. E. Yesalis, et al.
JAMA 270:1217-1221, 1993.
Reports on AAS use, characteristics, use of other illicit drugs, and relationship between AAS and aggressive behavior; data was obtained from
the 1991 National Household Survey on Drug Abuse (NHSDA).

Anabolic-androgenic steroids: prevalence, knowledge, and attitudes in junior and
senior high school students, by C. N. Luetkemeier, et al. JOURNAL OF
HEALTH EDUCATION 26(1):4-10, 1995.
Survey of junior and senior high school students in Utah to determine
AAS use, but also found more than half not aware of risks.

Anabolic steroid use among adolescents in a rural state, by R. Whitehead, et al.
JOURNAL OF FAMILY PRACTICE 35:401-405, 1992.
Study of 3900 male high school students in West Virginia found AAS
use associated with cigarette and illicit drug use; predominant reason was
to improve appearance. Prevalence was similar to metropolitan areas and
not related to size of school.

Anabolic steroid use among students at a British college of technology, by D. J.
Williamson. BRITISH JOURNAL OF SPORTS MEDICINE 27:200-201, 1993.
General survey of day students with a very high response rate of 92%
and further questions for AAS users; early use by males before age 17
for those who participated in bodybuilding, weight lifting or rugby. Variety
of students in both academic and practical courses were surveyed.

Anabolic steroid use, strength training and multiple drug use among adolescents
in the United States, by R. H. DuRant, et al. PEDIATRICS 96:23-28, 1995.
Report of a study of AAS use along with other drugs, sports performance, academic performance; statistics gathered from the 1991 CDC
Prevention Youth Risk Behavior Survey; confirmed polydrug use and
strength training.

Anabolic steroids: interest among parents and nonathletes, by P. S. Salva and G.
E. Bacon. SOUTHERN MEDICAL JOURNAL 84:552-556, 1991.
Physician survey in Texas to determine degree and extent of parental interest in AAS, particularly concerning football, but also for psychosocial
reasons; recommends that parents be included in prevention efforts to
decrease appropriate use.

Anabolic steroids: study of high school athletes, by C. B. Corbin, et al. PEDIATRIC
EXERCISE SCIENCE 6:149-158, 1994.
Study of a large sample of high school students to determine steroid use
rates and factors related to use; has implications for education efforts.

Anabolic use by adolescents: prevalence, motives, and knowledge of risks, by S.
Tanner, et al. JOURNAL OF SPORTS MEDICINE 5:108-115, 1995.
Study to determine prevalence of AAS use in Denver, Colorado by high
school students; assessed knowledge of risks and found many misconceptions, i.e. that AAS increase height; copy of questionnaire and references.

Androgenic anabolic steroid use in matric pupils, by M. P. Schwellnus, et al.
SOUTH AFRICAN MEDICAL JOURNAL 82:154-158, 1992.
Survey to determine prevalence of AAS use in Western Cape, South
Africa; general knowledge was poor about AAS use in . . . especially
among females and nonathletes; concludes that education is important
for school children.

Associations between academic performance of division 1 college athletes and their perceptions of the effects of anabolic steroids, by M. A. Perko, et al. PERCEPTUAL AND MOTOR SKILLS 80:284-286, 1995.

Authors compared the relationship between academic performance (GPA) and the perceptions of the effects of AAS and found that the lower the GPA, the more likely college athletes are to think that AAS improve performance and the less likely they are to think AAS are a threat to health. Authors recommend drug education that includes information about AAS.

Beliefs about steroids: user vs. nonuser comparisons, by M. J. Schwerin and K. J. Corcoran. DRUG AND ALCOHOL DEPENDENCE 40:221-225, 1996.

Results based on the beliefs about steroids scale (BASS) show that AAS users have greater beliefs in the effectiveness of AAS use than nonusers; AAS users expect positive results; statements from BASS are listed.

Characteristics of the elbow flexors in women bodybuilders using androgenic-anabolic steroids, by S. E. Alway. JOURNAL OF STRENGTH AND CONDITIONING RESEARCH 8(3):161-169, 1994.

A small sample of female AAS using bodybuilders was compared to nonusers and the AAS users were found to have greater lean body mass, greater hypertrophy of muscle fibers, less body fat, and experienced less fatigue. This is one of the few technical articles that reports a study of women and the author speculates that AAS may have a positive impact in sports that depend on high levels of muscle mass, body weight and strength.

Characteristics of steroid users in an adolescent school population, by E. M. Adlaf and R. G. Smart. JOURNAL OF ALCOHOL AND DRUG EDUCATION 38:43-49, 1992.

Reports on the rate of AAS use among Ontario students aged 13 to 19, demographics, sport involved with, perceived health status, and use of other drugs. Found lower use in Canada than US but some similarities.

Desire for weight gain and potential risks of adolescent males using anabolic steroids, by M. Q. Wang, et al. PERCEPTUAL AND MOTOR SKILLS 78: 267-274, 1994.

Provides current data from national sample on perceptions of adolescent boys regarding their physical strength, health, and desire to gain weight along with their perceptions of AAS use; high percentage of high school boys want to gain weight because of desired sports participation and thus are at risk for using AAS.

Despite warnings, lure of steroids too strong for some young Canadians, by S. Newman. CANADIAN MEDICAL ASSOCIATION JOURNAL 151:844-846, 1994.

Provides an overview of the data from a national survey on drugs and sport for Centre for Drug Free Sport, Canada; recent studies also reviewed.

Doping and high-level endurance walkers. Knowledge and representation of a prohibited practice, by P. Laure and H. Reinsberger. JOURNAL OF SPORTS MEDICINE AND PHYSICAL FITNESS 35:228-231, 1995.

Sample of male and female long distance walkers agree with drug testing, but disagree with the definition of doping in sport, i.e. analgesics should not be considered doping. Subjects were asked about general knowledge of substances, prevalence of use, etc.; using a self-reporting questionnaire.

Doping in Norwegian gyms—a big problem?, by N. A. Bergsgard, et al. INTERNATIONAL REVIEW FOR THE SOCIOLOGY OF SPORT 31:351-362, 1996.
>Authors did a survey and concluded that drug use is common in some gyms, but not a big problem in Norway. They compare their results with other surveys and recognize the limitations of surveys on sensitive topics and using indirect techniques.

Drug and alcohol use by Canadian university athletes: a national survey, by J. C. Spence and L. Gauvin. JOURNAL OF DRUG EDUCATION 26:275-287, 1996.
>Compiles self-reports of use and perceptions of the value of drug testing and education; steroids and cocaine reported less than American students.

Drug use among adolescent students in Canada and Ontario: past, present and future, by E. M. Adlaf and R. G. Smart. JOURNAL OF DRUG ISSUES 21:59-72, 1991.
>Discusses trends in multiple drug use in Ontario for which AAS were not included in this survey, but rather tobacco, alcohol, cannibis, heroin, LSD, cocaine, crack, etc.; some comparisons to U.S.

Drug use amongst young athletes, by R. R. Albrecht. SPORTS MEDICINE 22: 351-354, 1996.
>Author warns that terms are confusing and definitions unclear and not generalizable, i.e. what is a drug, what constitutes use, how old is young, and what makes a person an athlete?

Drugs, sex, and crime in sport: an Australian perspective, by M. Paccagnella and J. R. Grove. JOURNAL OF SPORT AND SOCIAL ISSUES 21:179-188, 1997.
>Authors investigated the impact of controversial publicity, including steroid use, on perceptions of well-known sport performers. Undergraduate students rated six high-profile sports stars and results showed that athletes associated with the use of performance-enhancing drugs were evaluated negatively. Steroid users were seen as dishonest and less rule-oriented than those convicted of crimes.

Dying to be big: a review of anabolic steroid use, by H. M. Perry, et al. BRITISH JOURNAL OF SPORTS MEDICINE 26:259-261, 1992.
>Results of a survey of private gymnasia users in Wales shows polydrug use to counteract AAS side effects and need for needle exchange program to reduce risk of HIV due to sharing needles.

Epidemiology and patterns of anabolic-androgenic steroid use, by C. E. Yesalis. PSYCHIATRIC ANNALS 22:7-18, 1992.
>"Adapted from ANABOLIC STEROIDS IN EXERCISE AND SPORT, Yesalis, C. E. (editor), Champaign, Illinois: Human Kinetics. Copyright 1992. . . ."

Gym and tonic: profile of 100 male steroid users, by N. A. Evans. BRITISH JOURNAL OF SPORTS MEDICINE 31:54-58, 1997.
>Results of a survey of athletes using four gymnasia; drugs used are listed and regimens discussed along with costs, adverse effects and withdrawal symptoms.

High-risk behaviors among high school students in Massachusetts who use anabolic steroids, by A. B. Middleman, et al. PEDIATRICS 96:268-272, 1995.
Report of AAS use based on the 1993 Youth Risk Behavior Survey; including tables and references.

Multimethod examination of the male anabolic steroid user, by M. J. Schwerin and K. J. Corcoran. JOURNAL OF APPLIED SOCIAL PSYCHOLOGY 26:211-217, 1996.
Examines perceptions of a male AAS user based on ratings of written descriptions; subjects viewed AAS users negatively.

Narcissism and empathy in steroid users, by J. H. Porcerelli and B. A. Sandler. AMERICAN JOURNAL OF PSYCHIATRY 152: 1672-1674, 1995.
Authors compared bodybuilders and weight lifters who did or did not use anabolic steroids on an objective measure of narcissism and clinical ratings of empathy.

Non-medical drug use behaviour at five U.S. universities: a 15-year study, by T. L. Dezelsky, et al. BULLETIN ON NARCOTICS 37:49-53, 1985.
Longitudinal survey carried out by questionnaire to observe trends in the use of cannabis, alcohol, cocaine, LSD, amphetamines, sedatives and anabolic steroids from 1970-1984.

Perceptions of anabolic steroid users, by J. L. Van Raalte, et al. JOURNAL OF APPLIED SOCIAL PSYCHOLOGY 23:1214-1225, 1993.
Use of steroid perception questionnaire (SPQ) to survey AS-using peer bodybuilders and found that users perceive fellow users positively. However, undergraduate nonusers see drug-using athletes as being like other drug users, thus view AS use negatively. Prevention is best aimed at populations at-risk.

Prevalence of anabolic steroid use among Illinois high school students, by G. L. Gaa, et al. JOURNAL OF ATHLETIC TRAINING 29:216-222, 1994.
Study to determine anabolic steroid use in Illinois, student knowledge, and characteristics of AAS user; over one third were non-athletes.

Rate of anabolic-androgenic steroid use among students in junior high school, by J. Radakovich, et al. JOURNAL OF THE AMERICAN BOARD OF FAMILY PRACTICE 6:341-345, 1993.
Study of seventh-grade students who completed a questionnaire about steroid use, knowledge of steroids; minorities and older students with past drug use were more likely to use.

Self-perceptions of the acute and long-range effects of anabolic-androgenic steroids, by L. J. Silvester. JOURNAL OF STRENGTH AND CONDITIONING RESEARCH 9:95-98, 1995.
Self-reports from twenty-two former athlete users showed that health problems were mostly nuisances rather than severe debilitating consequences; AAS use more of an ethical issue. Questions used are listed.

Sexual functioning of male anabolic steroid abusers, by H. B. Moss, et al. ARCHIVES OF SEXUAL BEHAVIOR 22:1-12, 1993.
Structured interviews were conducted with three different groups of bodybuilders: current users, past users ,and those who never used; current users had higher frequency of coital and orgasmic activity, but also erectile difficulties. Androgens appear to enhance sexual desire and appetite, but sexual assault not documented.

Social physique anxiety, body esteem, and social anxiety in bodybuilders and self-reported anabolic steroid users, by M. J. Schwerin, et al. ADDICTIVE BEHAVIORS 21:1-8, 1996.
Study of social physique anxiety (SPA), body esteem and related health problems in 185 AAS users and nonusers; AAS users have lower SPA and higher body strength and esteem and physical attractiveness.

Sociodemographic analysis of drug use among adolescent athletes: observations-perceptions of athletic directors-coaches, by E. W. Shields, Jr. ADOLESCENCE 30:839-861, 1995.
Examines substance abuse by high school athletes through the observations of athletic directors and coaches in North Carolina; suggests that participation in sports may deter drug abuse.

A survey of elite athletes on the perceived causes of using banned drugs in sport, by M. H. Anshel. JOURNAL OF SPORT BEHAVIOR 14:283-307, 1991.
Personal interviews were conducted with elite male and female athletes from the U.S. to investigate the causes of using performance enhancing and/or recreational or mind-altering drugs. Reasons differed for the two types. Data was grouped into three likely causes: physical, psychological/emotional and social. Examples of questions and sample quotes provided.

Use and awareness of effects of anabolic steroids and psychoactive substances among a cohort of Nigerian professional sports men and women, by J. U. Ohaeri, et al. HUMAN PSYCHOPHARMACOLOGY 8:429-432, 1993.
Nigerian drug-use rate among professional sports people screened for the Olympics was mostly lower but not much different from general population. Also seemed unaware of dangerous side effects of AAS . . . subject to peer pressure and those pushing use.

Use of anabolic-androgenic steroids among body builders—frequency and attitudes, by M. Lindström, et al. JOURNAL OF INTERNAL MEDICINE 227:407-411, 1990.
This reports on a survey of 138 male body builders, less than half had used AAS; questionnaire included. Blood pressure was not significantly different in users. Reported side effects listed and tallied.

The use of anabolic-androgenic steroids by Canadian students, by P. Melia, et al. CLINICAL JOURNAL OF SPORT MEDICINE 6:9-14, 1996.
Survey to establish baseline data on drug use of performance-enhancers by Canadian youth as well as knowledge and attitudes; 42 item questionnaire completed by students in schools across Canada regarding caffeine, AAS, beta-blockers, etc.; suspect under-reporting because of legal constraints; alarming relationship between AAS use, injection and sharing of needles, especially ages 11 to 13.

Use of anabolic steroids in high school students, by R. Terney and L. G. McLain. AMERICAN JOURNAL OF THE DISEASES OF CHILDREN 144:99-103, 1990.
Documents use of AAS among high school students in Chicago suburbs but may under-report; also general knowledge and awareness of side effects; sample of questionnaire included.

Use of multiple drugs among adolescents who use anabolic steroids, by R. H. DuRant, et al. NEW ENGLAND JOURNAL OF MEDICINE 328:922-926, 1993.

Surveyed 1881 students enrolled in compulsory high school health-science classes in Georgia; adolescent AAS users more likely to use other drugs, especially mood-altering, smokeless tobacco, marijuana, cocaine, etc., and that many share needles and risk HIV and other viral infections, believing they are at low risk.

What do people think of male steroid users? An experimental investigation, by M. J. Schwerin and K. J. Corcoran. JOURNAL OF APPLIED SOCIAL PSYCHOLOGY 22:833-840, 1992.

Using the steroid perception questionnaire, subjects from psychology classes were asked to rank the social desirability of a story protagonist: drug-free bodybuilder, steroid-using bodybuilder, cocaine-using bodybuilder; results reported that steroid and cocaine users viewed negatively.

Side Effects

This section is divided into physical and psychological effects that are associated with AAS use and related issues of the psychology of drug use, addiction or dependence, behavioral effects, body image, mood swings, violence and aggression. Physical effects include changes in the heart, liver, skin, blood lipids, hormones and impotence/infertility, HIV risk due to needle-sharing, and increased tendon injury. Psychological effects can include antisocial personality traits, body image disturbances, irritability, hostility, anxiety, decreased self-esteem, and depression. Many studies are based on self-reports. Some articles cover both physical and psychological effects but they have been sorted most appropriately.

Side Effects: Physical

An acute myocardial infarction occurring in an anabolic steroid user, by M. J. Huie. MEDICINE AND SCIENCE IN SPORTS AND EXERCISE 26:408-413, 1994.
> A case study is presented of an acute myocardial infarction occurring in an AAS user who was an amateur weight trainer, 25 year-old, with no prior medical history, but some family history of myocardial infarction; specific cause of coronary thrombosis was not clear but AAS may have been a factor.

Anabolic steroid-induced hypogonadotropic hypogonadism, by J. P. Jarow and L. I. Lipshultz. AMERICAN JOURNAL OF SPORTS MEDICINE 18:429-431, 1990.
> Provides two case reports of hypogonadism persisting for more than a year following discontinuation of AAS use; one patient was treated with human chorionic gonadotropin for infertility and the other patient complained of decreased libido and hormonal evaluation revealed a low serum testosterone concentration.

Anabolic steroid-induced tendon pathology: a review of the literature, by J. T. Laseter and J. A. Russell. MEDICINE AND SCIENCE IN SPORTS AND EXERCISE 23:1-3, 1991.
> Reviews animal studies on tendon pathology and AAS use and then applies these to humans with case reports linking tendon rupture.

Anabolic steroid use in body builders: an echocardiographic study of left ventricle morphology and function, by B. De Piccoli, et al. INTERNATIONAL JOURNAL OF SPORTS MEDICINE 12:408-412, 1991.
> Reports on a study of AAS using and nonusing bodybuilders; seems to show that AAS harm the myocardium, i.e. enlargement and thickening of the left ventricle.

Anabolic steroids and cardiovascular risk in athletes, by N. Nnakwe. NUTRITION TODAY 31(5):206-208, 1996.

    This article reviews the blood lipid abnormalities, high blood pressure, and the use of AAS as strong heart disease risk factors. Author concludes that based on research AAS cause detrimental changes in plasma lipid profile not buffered by the benefits of exercise.

Androgenic-anabolic steroid abuse and platelet aggregation: pilot study in weight-lifters, by G. S. Ferenchick, et al. AMERICAN JOURNAL OF THE MEDICAL SCIENCES 303(2):78-82, 1992.

    Suggests an association between androgen use, age, and increased platelet sensitivity to collagen; nonusers tested positive thus questioning subjective reporting when assessing androgen use among weightlifters.

Are 'roids really that dangerous?, by J. Antonio. JOE WEIDER'S MUSCLE AND FITNESS, November 1996, pp. 110-112+.

    Interview with researcher Antonio who says that the serious risks of anabolic androgenic steroids are greatly exaggerated. Side effects are reversible or minor and few deaths could clearly be associated with the use of AAS alone.

Association of anabolic steroids and avascular necrosis of femoral heads, by K. A. Pettine. AMERICAN JOURNAL OF SPORTS MEDICINE 19:96-98, 1991.

    A patient and former AAS user reported two years of increasing hip pain and was found to have decreased range of motion in the hips. He had to use crutches and have repeated surgeries.

Atherogenic effects of anabolic steroids on serum lipid levels, by G. Glazer. ARCHIVES OF INTERNAL MEDICINE 151:1925-1933, 1991.

    Review article on the current body of literature on AAS and atherogenic changes in serum lipid levels and thus increased risk of coronary heart disease due to AAS use. Technical review with much detail, but overall total cholesterol levels not significantly changed during AAS use. Liver and heart problems seem to be due to oral AAS.

Athletes on anabolic-androgenic steroids, by M. Frankle and D. Leffers. PHYSICIAN AND SPORTS MEDICINE 20(6):75-76+, June 1992.

    Two orthopedic physicians offered a steroid clinic with laboratory testing for potential health problems, lengthy interview, and physical exam. Idea was to discourage or reduce use but not to judge. Most with some significant medical problems returned to reduce side effects. Patient demographics charted.

Bigger, faster, stronger?, by C. Siff. FITNESS AND SPORTS REVIEW INTERNATIONAL 29:23-25, 1994.

    Questions current strength training methods but warns of increased injuries to muscles, tendons and ligaments by the abuse of AAS.

Bilateral rupture of the quadriceps tendon associated with anabolic steroids, by R. Y. L. Liow and S. Tavares. BRITISH JOURNAL OF SPORTS MEDICINE 29: 77-79, 1995.

    Reports a case of a 29-year-old bodybuilder whose AAS use appeared to predispose him to tendon rupture in both knees.

Cardiotoxic effects of cocaine and AAS in the athlete, by A. A. Welder and R. B. Melchert. JOURNAL OF PHARMACOLOGICAL AND TOXICOLOGICAL METHODS 29:61-68, 1993.
> Overview of AAS cardiotoxicity and technical review that tries to prove that AAS have a negative impact on exercise and that abusers of cocaine or AAS are at risk for myocardial infarction due to adverse effects. Authors cite ER episodes and deaths of several athletes and case reports.

Cardiovascular effects of anabolic steroids, by R. C. Becker and J. Ansell. PRIMARY CARDIOLOGY 20:26-27+, 1994.
> This is a brief article that reviews several studies that point to adverse venous and arterial thrombotic events due to AAS use. Low testosterone level appears to be a risk factor for ischemic heart disease.

Cardiovascular effects of androgenic-anabolic steroids, by R. B. Melchert and A. A. Welder. MEDICINE AND SCIENCE IN SPORTS AND EXERCISE 27:1252-1262, 1995.
> Authors present four models of AAS-induced adverse cardiovascular effects using what evidence has accumulated so far based on case studies and experimental animal studies. Technical article with extensive references.

Cardiovascular implications of anabolic steroid abuse, by K. Cheever and M. A. House. JOURNAL OF CARDIOVASCULAR NURSING 6(2):19-30, 1992.
> Explains heart side effects, symptoms, and nursing implications for history-taking, for example, sheet of guidelines with specific questions provided.

Chromosome investigations in weightlifter and powerlifters after intake of anabolic steroids, by L. Pysny and N. Hola. SPORTS MEDICINE, TRAINING AND REHABILITATION 4:15-19, 1993.
> Technical article reports results of blood samples from weightlifters/ powerlifters who answered positively to taking AAS (17/231) for longer than 3 months; these were analyzed for genotoxic risk for malignant diseases. Concern reported for HIV/AIDS because most took AAS in form of injections. Table shows correlation between aberrant cells and AAS use.

Echocardiography in fraternal twin bodybuilders with one abusing anabolic steroids, by R. D. Dickerman, et al. CARDIOLOGY 88:50-51, 1997.
> This is a letter to the editor reporting on a study of twin bodybuilders, one had used anabolic steroids for 15 years and the other remained steroid free, suggests that AAS may cause left ventricular hypertrophy without affecting cardiac function.

Effects of anabolic-androgenic steroids on the pilosebaceous unit, by M. J. Scott, III and A. M. Scott. CUTIS 50(2):113-116, August 1, 1992.
> Reviews the skin side effects as a result of using AAS: acne, oily hair and skin, cysts, increased body hair, loss of scalp hair, etc. Technical terms are used throughout and skin biopsy specimens illustrated.

The effects of anabolic steroids on myocardial structure and cardiovascular fitness, by T. R. Sachtleben, et al. MEDICINE AND SCIENCE IN SPORTS AND EXERCISE 25:1240-1245, 1993.
> Researchers studied myocardial structure, maximum oxygen consumption and body composition in steroid-using weight trainers while off cycle and again at the peak of a cycle. Chronic effects were also studied by comparing weight trainer-users off cycle with those who had no history of steroid use.

The efficacy of ergogenic agents in athletic competition. Part 1: androgenic-anabolic steroids, by D. A. Smith and P. J. Perry. ANNALS OF PHARMA-COTHERAPY 26:520-528, 1992.
Summarizes the epidemiology, pharmacology, and adverse effects associated with AAS use; 88 references.

Endocrine effects in female weight lifters who self-administer testosterone and anabolic steroids, by W. B. Malarkey, et al. AMERICAN JOURNAL OF OBSTETRICS AND GYNECOLOGY 165:1385-1390, 1991.
One of the very few studies that investigates the endocrine effects of AAS on females; AAS users reported menstrual irregularities, and other side effects. Users also had lower HDL cholesterol levels and may be at risk for developing heart disease.

Extreme hyperbilirubinemia associated with the use of anabolic steroids, health/nutritional supplements, and ethanol: response to ursodeoxycholic acid treatment, by C. Singh, et al. AMERICAN JOURNAL OF GASTROENTEROLOGY 91(4):783-785, 1996.
Case study presented of a young male bodybuilder, AAS user with profound jaundice; patient also drank a case of beer per day and used herbal and nutritional supplements.

Impotence related to anabolic steroid use in a body builder response to clomiphene citrate, by C. Bickelman, et al. WESTERN JOURNAL OF MEDICINE 162:158-160, 1995.
Case report of a 29-year-old man who had impotence and decreased libido for a year; clomiphene used to treat pituitary-gonadal failure.

Influence of anabolic steroids on body composition, blood pressure, lipid profile and liver functions in body builders, by H. Kuipers, et al. INTERNATIONAL JOURNAL OF SPORTS MEDICINE 12:413-418, 1991.
Study of the effects of AAS on bodybuilders (some received placebo) showed the AAS caused a decrease in HDL-cholesterol which was reversed after cessation of drug use; also AAS caused an increase in blood pressure; but no harmful effects on liver enzymes noted; and lean body mass was superior for AAS users.

Intramuscular abscess, by C. Maropis and E. Yesalis. PHYSICIAN AND SPORTS MEDICINE 22(10):105-108, October 1994.
Case report of a 24-year-old male who developed an abscess after re-using needles to inject anabolic-androgenic steroids; warns that needle-sharing can lead to hepatitis or HIV.

Left ventricular function is not impaired in weight-lifters who use anabolic steroids, by P. D. Thompson, et al. JOURNAL OF THE AMERICAN COLLEGE OF CARDIOLOGY 19:278-282, 1992.
Urine testing required as athletes who use AAS frequently do not know true identity of drugs; failed to document differences in cardiac function between AAS users and nonusers.

Let doctors manage steroids, by A. Millar. MODERN MEDICINE OF AUSTRALIA 38:128-131, 1995.
Refutes the harmful effects reported and recommends doctor supervised approach called, harm reduction programme.

Linear keloids resulting from abuse of anabolic androgenic steroid drugs, by M. J. Scott, et al. CUTIS 53:41-43, January 1994.

Report of three case studies of rare skin enlargement over striated muscle due to AAS use; recommended discontinuing AAS use so no new lesions; commentary on random test results and false negatives.

Multiple HIV-risk behaviors among injection-steroid users, by D. D. Lenaway, et al. AIDS AND PUBLIC POLICY JOURNAL 7:184-186, 1992.

Describes a syringe-and-needle-exchange program for cocaine, heroin, speed, but also injection-steroid users (ISUs) who do not always use condoms during sex and thus expose themselves and others to HIV and/or hepatitis B. Authors encourage wider implementation of outreach programs designed for ISUs, who do not see themselves at high risk for HIV.

Myocardial infarction associated with anabolic steroid use in a previously healthy 37-year-old weightlifter, by G. S. Ferenchick and S. Adelmen. AMERICAN HEART JOURNAL 124(2):507-508, August 1992.

Case study reported of weightlifter with history of AAS use over seven years and ingested up to twenty aspirins per day for chronic headaches; reports elevated serum cholesterol levels frequently in athletes who use androgens.

Parade's guide to better fitness, by M. O'Shea. PARADE MAGAZINE May 24, 1992, pp. 34-35.

Q&A format about Lyle Alzado who died of a brain tumor and believed his steroid use was the cause; briefly reviews harmful side effects.

Peliosis hepatis in a young adult bodybuilder, by A. Cabasso. MEDICINE AND SCIENCE IN SPORTS AND EXERCISE 26(1):2-4, 1994.

Case report of a 27-year-old male bodybuilder who developed rare condition of blood-filled sacs in the liver after chronic use of anabolic steroids; extensive references.

Resistance trained athletes using or not using anabolic steroids compared to runners: effects on cardiorespiratory variables, body composition, and plasma lipids, by R. Yeater, et al. BRITISH JOURNAL OF SPORTS MEDICINE 30:11-14, 1996.

Concludes that resistance training without AAS results in the same positive effects on cardiac size and functions as aerobic training.

Serum lipids, lipoproteins, electrolytes, and urinary creatinine and electrolytes excretion in anabolic steroids user and nonusers on self-selected diets, by N. Nnakwe. SPORTS MEDICINE, TRAINING AND REHABILITATION 3:271-279, 1992.

No significant differences found between AAS user and nonusers in terms of serum lipids; suggests that low-fat diet in users may alleviate negative influence of AAS use.

Serum lipoprotein patterns in long-term anabolic steroid users, by T. R. Sachtleben, et al. RESEARCH QUARTERLY FOR EXERCISE AND SPORT 68:110-115, 1997.

Study compared AAS users and nonusers and determined that AAS users, even with 8-12 weeks of nonuse, are at risk for early atherosclerosis due to harmful effects on serum lipids; reviews and compares with selected other studies.

Steroid roulette. WOMEN'S SPORTS AND FITNESS 14:18-19, October 1992.
Examines risks for female AAS users; covers how they work, side effects, benefits, emotions affected, and sample cases.

Steroids and sports are a losing proposition, by R. Mishra. FDA CONSUMER 25:24-27, 1991.
Reports three case studies of steroid uses and the negative consequences and explains newer trends in the use of alternatives such as: GHB, clenbuterol, etc.

Steroids: what you have to lose, by R. Dinsmoor. CURRENT HEALTH 2 20:22-24, February 1994.
Briefly reviews potential side effects, both physical and psychological.

Sudden cardiac death during exercise in a weight lifter using anabolic androgenic steroids: pathological and toxicological findings, by J. L. Luke, et al. JOURNAL OF FORENSIC SCIENCES 35:1441-1447, 1990.
Case report of a 21-year-old weightlifter who died suddenly during a bench press workout with the possible cause being AAS use.

Use of anabolic steroids by athletes, by J. R. Bierly. POSTGRADUATE MEDICINE 82:67-74, 1987.
Reviews the side effects, especially liver and cardiovascular.

What determines strength?, by M. Yessis. FITNESS AND SPORTS REVIEW INTERNATIONAL 27:8-9, 1992.
Reviews and lists the major factors that determine strength of muscles; use of AAS produces bulk, but increases injury.

Side Effects: Psychological

Aggression and hostility in anabolic steroid users, by W. R. Yates, et al. BIOLOGICAL PSYCHIATRY 31:1232-1234, 1992.
Although aggressive and violent behaviors appear to be linked to anabolic steroid use, it was impossible for these researchers to determine if aggressive effects occurred prior to AAS use; high prevalence of antisocial personality traits may be present in AAS users.

Aggression, the law and anabolic steroid users, by H. M. Perry. NEW LAW JOURNAL 143:1742-1743, December 10, 1993.
This is a brief overview and reporting of some of the violent side effects of AAS, especially very potent veterinary drugs which are highly androgenic.

Anabolic-androgenic steroid use-abuse (in males) progression chart, by M. J. Minelli, et al. ADDICTION AND RECOVERY 11:14-16, 1991.
Includes detailed table of symptoms progression from the early to middle to late stages of steroid abuse.

Anabolic-androgenic steroid use among male gymnasium participants: dependence, knowledge and motives, by D. W. Gridley and S. J. Hanrahan. SPORT HEALTH 12:11-14, 1994.
Good brief readable article about psychological side effects using the DSM III R criterion symptoms categorized by self-reported symptoms and statements of reasons for use; authors found body size dissatisfaction

among users, particularly dependent users. (DSM=DIAGNOSTIC AND STATISTICAL MANUAL OF MENTAL DISORDERS)

Anabolic-androgenic steroids and psychiatric-related effects [a review], by L. Uzych. CANADIAN JOURNAL OF PSYCHIATRY 37:23-27, 1992.
Good overview of the adverse psychiatric and behavioral effects, including episodes of mania, aggression, depression, etc., but more reliable studies needed to verify clinical observations. Testosterone propionate has been shown to increase erectile capacity and the strength of the sex drive, but AAS have a negative effect on the libido. Many studies used small samples and thus are of limited significance.

Anabolic steroid use by amateur athletes: effects upon psychological mood states, by A. C. Parrott, et al. JOURNAL OF SPORTS MEDICINE AND PHYSICAL FITNESS 34:292-298, 1994.
Twenty-one male amateur athletes completed two questionnaires about feelings. They were part of a Welsh needle-exchange program. They reported higher degrees of aggression, hostility, irritability, anxiety, negativism, etc. while on steroids.

Androgenic-anabolic steroids and body dysmorphic in young men, by A. Wroblewska. JOURNAL OF PSYCHOSOMATIC RESEARCH 42:225-234, 1997.
Review studies that have suggested social and psychological factors in AAS use, but says that controlled studies are clearly lacking; good overview of history, side effects, and discussion of possible body image and social pressure reasons for AAS use; 75 references.

Anger and aggression in women: influence of sports choice and testosterone administration, by S. Van Goozen, et al. AGGRESSIVE BEHAVIOR 20:213-222, 1994.
Sport choice did not reflect a difference in anger proneness, but androgen administration does increase anger proneness.

Anorexia nervosa and "reverse anorexia" among 108 male bodybuilders, by H. G. Pope, et al. COMPREHENSIVE PSYCHIATRY 34:406-409, 1993.
Describes a disorder among young male weightlifters who see themselves as too small despite being large and muscular. This disorder of body image may contribute to the misuse of AAS in some individuals. Data was based on a study of bodybuilders in Massachusetts and California and four case report examples are described.

Assessing the threat of anabolic steroids, by D. Catlin, et al. PHYSICIAN AND SPORTS MEDICINE 21:37-44, 1993.
Interview Q&A format is used with four medical experts in the use of AAS; covers use, testing, masking, how obtained, effects, counseling, substitutes, reverse anorexia nervosa, etc.

Assessment of attentional bias and mood in users and non-users of anabolic-androgenic steroids, by A. J. Bond, et al. DRUG AND ALCOHOL DEPENDENCE 37:241-245, 1995.
Strength athletes were studied for attentional bias to aggressive clues, but no significant differences were found between current, former or nonusers of AAS. Current steroid use produced subtle mood changes.

Body image and steroid use in male bodybuilders, by A. G. Blouin and G. S.
Goldfield. INTERNATIONAL JOURNAL OF EATING DISORDERS 18:159-
165, 1995.
Examined whether AAS use was associated with body image disturbances in athletes; bodybuilders reported greater body dissatisfaction
and lower self-esteem and the greatest use of AAS.

A case of affective disorder associated with the misuse of "anabolic steroids," by
H. M. Perry and G. W. Hughes. BRITISH JOURNAL OF SPORTS MEDICINE
26:219-220, 1992.
Brief report of an AAS user seen by a psychiatrist for severe acute depression and suicidal ideas after the use of haldol decanoate and an appetite stimulant; suggests that AAS users have little knowledge of the
substances they are injecting.

A high prevalence of abnormal personality traits in chronic uses of anabolic-
androgenic steroids, by C. J. Cooper, et al. BRITISH JOURNAL OF SPORTS
MEDICINE 30:246-250, 1996.
Participant-observation used to determine if bodybuilder AAS users
showed signs of abnormal personality traits and the results suggest that
AAS use is associated with personality disturbances.

Homicide and near-homicide by anabolic steroid users, by H. G. Pope and D. L.
Katz. JOURNAL OF CLINICAL PSYCHIATRY 51(1):28-31, 1990.
Presents three case histories which raise the suspicion of steroid-
induced violence in otherwise nonviolent individuals who exhibited no
previous evidence of antisocial behavior and yet who committed violent
crimes, including murder, while under the influence of AAS.

Illicit anabolic steroid use: a controlled personality study, by W. R. Yates, et al.
ACTA PSYCHIATRICA SCANDINAVIA 81(6):548-550, 1990.
Illicit AAS users demonstrated significant antisocial traits which were
common to both alcoholics and AAS users; the AAS users were weightlifters and all participants responded using a self-report measure.

Illicit anabolic steroid use in athletes: a case series analysis, by P. J. Perry, et al.
AMERICAN JOURNAL OF SPORTS MEDICINE 18:422-428, 1990.
Steroid use histories of twenty weightlifters were examined to find that
AAS users take both oral and injectable drugs. Subjects reported gains
in body weight and strength and mental status changes, i.e. symptoms of
depression, hostility, aggression and paranoia.

Indications of psychological dependence among anabolic-androgenic steroid
abusers, by C. E. Yesalis, et al. NATIONAL INSTITUTE ON DRUG ABUSE
RESEARCH MONOGRAPH SERIES 102:196-213, 1990.
Chapter adapted from earlier article, "Anabolic Steroid use," JOURNAL
OF DRUG EDUCATION 19:1031-116, 1989.

Neuropsychiatric effects of anabolic steroids in male normal volunteers, by T.-P.
Su, et al. JAMA 269(21):2760-2764, 1993.
Study of behavioral effects of anabolic steroids; confirmed increased
hostility, anxiety, depression, but also heightened energy.

An overview of sport psychiatry, by D. Begel. AMERICAN JOURNAL OF
PSYCHIATRY 149:606-614, 1992.
This is an interesting and very well-referenced paper that provides an historical overview and philosophical discussion of a field that needs more
research. Drug abuse and specifically anabolic steroid abuse are men-

tioned briefly as promoting aggressive behavior, but also that behavior therapies can enhance athletic performance. The author speculates that a psychiatrist who is a sports fan might prescribe controlled substances in the interest of improving a patient's performance.

Personality, mood and psychiatric symptoms among anabolic steroid users, by H. B. Moss, et al. AMERICAN JOURNAL OF ADDICTIONS 1:315-324, 1992.
No personality differences noted between AAS users and nonusers except for a tendency toward increased aggression and hostility among users.

Personality profile of men using anabolic androgenic steroids, by N. Galligani, et al. HORMONES AND BEHAVIOR 30:170-175, 1996.
Reviews animal and human behavior studies and then reports on a study of personality traits in three groups of strength athletes; subjects completed the Karolinska Scales of Personality, measuring traits related to anxiety, aggression, hostility and extroversion. Confirmed that AAS use is associated with enhanced aggressiveness. Also makes some comparisons with male alcoholics.

Psychiatric and medical effects of anabolic-androgenic steroid use, by H. G. Pope and D. L. Katz. ARCHIVES OF GENERAL PSYCHIATRY 51:375-382, 1994.
High dose steroid users displayed major mood syndromes, including mania, major depression, and sometimes violent behavior.

Psychiatric effects and psychoactive substance use in anabolic-androgenic steroid users, by D. A. Malone, et al. CLINICAL JOURNAL OF SPORT MEDICINE 5:25-31, 1995.
User categories did not differ significantly on psychological testing, but past AAS users had higher incidence of psychiatric diagnosis than nonuser and current user. Major depression followed AAS discontinuation. Psychoactive substance abuse was low in all groups.

Psychiatric effects of anabolic steroids, by H. G. Pope and D. L. Katz. PSYCHIATRIC ANNALS 22(1):24-29, 1992.
This is a good overview of studies and methods/tools used, i.e. Structured Clinical Interview (DSM-III-R) and Multi-Dimensional Anger Inventory (MDAI), concerning psychological effects of AAS on bodybuilders, football players, etc. Also makes some comparisons with corticosteroids which have been known to produce affective and psychotic symptoms. Steroid withdrawal may cause depressive symptoms and may contribute to dependence.

Psychiatric symptoms associated with anabolic steroids: controlled, retrospective study, by P. J. Perry, et al. ANNALS OF CLINICAL PSYCHIATRY 2:11-17, 1990.
There are mild/minor reactions not major mental disorders reported.

Psychoactive drugs and athletic performance, by T. L. Schwenk. PHYSICIAN AND SPORTS MEDICINE 25:32-34+, 1997.
Discusses the physiology of psychoactive drugs (otc and recreational and prescription) and what they are used for in terms of therapy and ergogenic effects; warns physicians to be aware of deliberate or unintentional use and their side effects in young athletes.

Psychological and behavioral effects of endogenous testosterone and anabolic-androgenic steroids [an update], by M. S. Bahrke, et al. SPORTS MEDICINE 22(6):367-390, December 1, 1996.
    Very thorough review of articles on the mental effects of testosterone and AAS abuse; reviews history and use and cites 157 references.

Psychological and behavioral effects of endogenous testosterone levels and anabolic-androgenic steroids among males [a review], by M. S. Bahrke, et al. SPORTS MEDICINE 10:303-337, 1990.
    Overview article covering the history, effects, therapy, mental health, behavior, psychological dependence, prevention and treatment of AAS abuse, research methods, etc.

Psychological and serum homovanillic acid changes in men administered androgenic steroids, by C. J. Hannan, et al. PSYCHONEUROENDOCRINOLOGY 16(4):335-343, 1991.
    Thirty healthy young (under age 40) active-duty military men were administered weekly injections of testosterone enanthate or nandrolone decanoate, 100 or 300 mg; subjects answered questions from the MMPI before and after androgen administration. Psychomotor task performance was compared between low and high dose and between the two different androgens.

Psychological characteristics of adolescent steroid users, by K. F. Burnett and M. E. Kleinman. ADOLESCENCE 29(113):81-88, Spring 1994.
    No personality characteristics found to be statistically significant between adolescent users and nonusers, but steroid users currently on a cycle had higher levels of depression, anger, mood changes, etc. than those not on a cycle. Negative physical side effects also reported by users.

Psychological moods and subjectively perceived behavioral and somatic changes accompanying anabolic-androgenic steroid use in male weight lifters, by M. S. Bahrke and J. E. Wright. AMERICAN JOURNAL OF SPORTS MEDICINE 20(6):717-724, November 1992.
    Assesses and discusses both physiological changes and psychological mood states with AAS use.

Psychological treatment of anabolic-androgenic steroid-dependent individuals, by J. P. Corcoran and E. Longo. JOURNAL OF SUBSTANCE ABUSE TREATMENT 9:229-235, 1992.
    Overview article that compares AAS use with cocaine and eating disorders and body image issues; suggests positive self-talk, imagery, relaxation, group treatment for AAS-dependent individual recovery.

Raging bull: the real dope on how steroids affect your mind, by J. Wright. JOE WEIDER'S MUSCLE AND FITNESS, February 1996, pp. 137-138+.
    This is an excellent overview article on the known facts about psychological side effects of taking AAS, including positive changes and possible dependence. Wright is an expert and says that the negative and violent and depressive effects have been overstated, but there has been some evidence of dependence.

Relationship between anabolic steroid use and selected psychological parameters in male bodybuilders, by R. G. Lefavi, et al. JOURNAL OF SPORT BEHAVIOR 13:157-166, 1990.
    Concludes that AAS use be associated with more frequent anger, hostility, sometimes along with violence and lack of control; results based on self-reports of male bodybuilders.

Roid rage: anabolic steroid use is exploding—with shattering consequences, by O. Fultz. AMERICAN HEALTH May 1991, pp. 60-65.
Covers use, side effects, withdrawal symptoms, etc.

Social psychobiologic dysfunction associated with anabolic steroid abuse [a review], by E. Gregg and W. J. Rejeski. SPORT PSYCHOLOGIST 4:275-284, 1990.
Reviews both human and nonhuman primate research and anecdotal reports of psychological effects; also reviews evidence for cardiovascular disease risk and potential for dependence or addiction.

Steroids: when pumping up can lead to serious health problems and side effects, by C. M. Groark. PREVENTION PIPELINE 5(1):83-85, January/February 1992 (reprinted from EMPLOYEE ASSISTANCE: Solutions to the Problems 4(4):8, November 1991).
Covers briefly who uses, history, availability, black market publications, side effects, possible addiction, parent and student education.

Three cases of nalbuphine hydrochloride dependence associated with anabolic steroid use, by A. J. McBride, et al. BRITISH JOURNAL OF SPORTS MEDICINE 30:69-70, 1996.
Reports opioid dependence for treatment of pain suffered by AAS users; nalbuphine is available on the black market and AAS users use to overcome musculoskeletal pain, despite risk of injury, to keep calm before competing, and to continue to train after injury.

Treating steroid abuse: a psychiatric perspective, by A. J. Giannini, et al. CLINICAL PEDIATRICS 30:538-542, 1991.
Provides a good overview of detection, treatment, prevalence and patterns of use, addiction and withdrawal and detoxification, self-help and addiction groups.

The use of anabolic-androgenic steroids (AAS) in sport and physical activity [a position statement], by The International Society of Sport Psychology. INTERNATIONAL JOURNAL OF SPORT PSYCHOLOGY 24(1):74-78, 1993.
Reviews the research concerning AAS use; supports the prohibition of AAS use by athletes due to the negative effects.

Use of fluoxetine in depression associated with anabolic steroid withdrawal [a case series], by D. A. Malone. JOURNAL OF CLINICAL PSYCHIATRY 53:130-132, 1992.
Anabolic steroid withdrawal depression was successfully treated with fluoxetine (prozac) and authors warn that the length of depression in these four case studies suggests that AAS withdrawal may precipitate the onset of major depression.

Violence toward women and illicit androgenic-anabolic steroid use, by P. Y. L. Choi and H. G. Pope. ANNALS OF CLINICAL PSYCHIATRY 6(1):21-25, 1994.
Study that found more reported fights, verbal aggression and violence toward a significant other for AAS users when they were on-cycle as opposed to off-cycle. This was based on self-reported data. High doses of several AAS related to violent behavior and examples are given of instances. A follow-up study of the wives and girlfriends would prove useful to verify self-reports.

Weight training: a potential confounding factor in examining the psychological and behavioral effects of anabolic-androgenic steroids, by M. S. Bahrke and C. E. Yesalis. SPORTS MEDICINE 18:309-318, 1994.
Thorough review article considers AAS and dependence along with weight training, mood, and self-esteem; suggests that psychological changes are a result of several factors that include restrictive diet and intensive training for AAS-using bodybuilders; 80 references.

Testing, Drug Enforcement, and Legal Studies

This section includes articles on doping control, drug testing, illegal black market, drug abuse enforcement, banned drugs, detection or screening methods used and proposed, policies and position statements, agreements and laws. A separate subsection on the Fourth and Fourteenth Amendments of the U.S. Constitution, privacy, search and seizure, and drug testing of college and public school athletes, includes articles on the controversial 1995 Vernonia v. Acton Supreme Court decision which upheld the random suspicionless mass drug testing of elementary, junior and senior public high school student athletes.

The abuse of doping agents in competing bodybuilders in Flanders (1988-1993), by F. T. Delbeke, et al. INTERNATIONAL JOURNAL OF SPORTS MEDICINE 16:66-70, 1995.
> Reports the result of a Belgium study of unannounced doping control which discovered widespread polydrug use, including AAS, testosterone, and clenbuterol.

Anabolic-androgenic steroid use by athletes. NATIONAL STRENGTH AND CONDITIONING ASSOCIATION JOURNAL 15(2):9 1993.
> This is a position statement with ten parts, covering the use of AAS as illegal and promoting athletic performance based on proper training methods and fair play.

Anabolic-androgenic steroid use by soldiers: U.S. Army steroid testing policy, by M. S. Bahrke and J. S. O'Connor. MILITARY MEDICINE 155:573-574, 1990.
> Brief article concluded that testing is not necessary because only occasional use.

Anabolic steroid and human growth hormone abuse: creating an effective and equitable ergogenic drug policy, by G. Fan. UNIVERSITY OF CHICAGO LEGAL FORUM 1994, pp. 439-470.
> Reviews the clinical uses of steroids and HGH, history of use, Anabolic Steroids Control Act of 1990 and comments on the failure to impose criminal sanctions on the use of HGH along with AAS.

The Anabolic Steroids Control Act of 1990: a need for change, by J. A. Black. DICKINSON LAW REVIEW 97:131-152, Fall 1992.
> Explains the legislation, historical background, previous state and federal legislation, purpose and intent.

Anabolic steroids: the price of pumping up!, by N. M. Reddig. WAYNE LAW REVIEW 37:1647-1682, 1990-1991.
> This is a very thorough and extensive overview of the use of AAS by adolescents, anabolic steroid defense, NFL policy, NCAA policy, state and federal legislation, penalties for coaches and trainers promoting

AAS, current illegal status and black market, and education aimed at preventing use. Numerous legal references are cited, including hearings,
cases, and a government study and also detailed footnotes.

The ban on drugs in sports, by T. Black and A. Pape. JOURNAL OF SPORT AND
SOCIAL ISSUES 21:83-92, 1997.
Authors argue that the removal of a ban on drugs will result in fair contests
and that athletes would benefit from medical advice. They also report that
there is a need for knowledge of safe dosages and standard products
commercially available at low-cost.

Beating drug tests, by M. G. Di Pasquale. DRUGS IN SPORTS 1(2):3-6, 1992.
Explains technical measurements such as T/E ratio used to detect ex-
ogenous testosterone and the potential inaccuracy and continuing controversy over masking agents, etc.

The big push: federal prosecutors pump iron into their campaign against bodybuilding steroids, by R. Sherman. NATIONAL LAW JOURNAL February 10,
1992, pp. 40+.
Reporting of drug abuse enforcement efforts (Duchaine prosecuted)
concerning counterfeit drugs; suggests clenbuterol be added to controlled substances act; and that more successful cases prosecuted because of the Anabolic Steroids Control Act.

Black-market biotechnology: athletes abuse EPO and hGH, by B. J. Spalding.
BIOTECHNOLOGY 9:1050+, 1991.
FDA warns that hGH on the black-market is not the real thing, i.e. counterfeit, but far less available than AAS, indicating less use. EPO's advantage
is that it is not detectable because natural cannot be distinguished from
recombinant and makers refuse to modify because of possible immune
response in anemia patients. People are very cautious about EPO because the information is out that it can kill.

Book reviews: Navigating the Yellow Stream, by K. A. Manson. MILITARY LAW
REVIEW 139:201-203, Winter 1993.
Author gives a poor review of the book about beating a drug test, saying
that the book contains misinformation and no scientific data. Author also
reviews the steps to an effective drug testing program.

Centennial Olympic Games, by R. L. Worsnop. CQ RESEARCHER 6:291-298,
April 5, 1996.
Drug detection and drug abuse are discussed as being linked to the
commercialism and professionalism of Olympic sport. There is some discussion of banned drug and testing methods as well as those substances for which no reliable test has been devised: HGH and EPO.

China drug bust, by P. Whitten. SWIMMING WORLD AND JUNIOR SWIMMER
36(1):71+, 1995.
Another in a series of reports on China's drug abuse testing woes;
Chinese swimmers had abnormally high levels of testosterone.

China drug controversy, by P. Whitten. SWIMMING WORLD AND JUNIOR SWIM-
MER 35:29, February 1994.
One-page description of the Chinese coaching methods with recom-
mendations regarding testing for EPO in the blood rather than urine.

China ousted from Pan Pacific Championships, by P. Whitten. SWIMMING WORLD AND JUNIOR SWIMMER 36:31-32, March 1995.
Reports that China was barred from the Pan Pacific Championships due to overwhelming evidence that China engaged in systematic doping of its athletes. DHT was the substance found in all but one of the 38 (10 swimmers and 28 in several different sports). FINA has been slow to respond say U.S., Canada and Australia.

China's short march to swimming dominance: hard work or drugs?, by P. Whitten. SWIMMING WORLD AND JUNIOR SWIMMER 35:34-39, January 1994.
Compares the success of Chinese female swimmers to the East Germans before 1989; EPO, HGH, and steroids discussed as well as comments from other top swimmers that accuse the Chinese of illegal drug use and cheating.

Chinese secrets, by M. C. Siff. FITNESS AND SPORTS REVIEW INTERNATIONAL 28:109-111, 1993.
Editorial and commentary that Americans are quick to rush to the conclusion of drug abuse rather than learn from Russian and Chinese training methods.

Chinese takeout, by C. Lord. SWIMMING WORLD AND JUNIOR SWIMMER 35: 60-69, November 1994.
Discusses the power of the Chinese women swimmers at Rome World Championships, taking each day from one to six, with illustrations; records and results listed for all events, including diving. Chinese had phenomenal starts and turns.

Clinical assessment and urine testing for anabolic-androgenic steroid abuse and dependence, by K. J. Brower, et al. AMERICAN JOURNAL OF DRUG AND ALCOHOL ABUSE 17:161-171, 1991.
Reviews the assessment of steroid abuse and dependence and the role of urine testing, illustrating with case studies.

Danger in the locker room, by L. Wolf. BUFFALO PHYSICIAN AND BIOMEDICAL SCIENTIST 25:21-23, 1991.
Researchers presenting papers at an international congress on psychoneuroendocrinology urge increased drug testing and research into alternative training methods and rehabilitation for addicted athletes. This is a brief overview of papers presented and review of previous research.

Detection in blood and urine of recombinant erythropoietin administered to healthy men, by L. Wide, et al. MEDICINE AND SCIENCE IN SPORTS AND EXERCISE 27:1569-1576, 1995.
DNA-recombinant EPO is classed as a doping substance, but no methods have been devised for testing; authors determine that injections of rhEPO can be detected 24 to 48 hours after injection, but not one week later. Further development is needed for doping control.

The determination of anabolic steroids by MECC, gradiant HPLC, and capillary GC, by I. S. Lurie, et al. JOURNAL OF FORENSIC SCIENCES 39:74-85, 1994.
This is a very technical article presenting methodologies for qualitative/quantitative determination of AAS. Numerous charts and tables document the results and analyses.

Doped to perfection, by G. Cowley, et al. NEWSWEEK 128:31+, July 22, 1996.
Good overview on testing developments, variety of drugs used that are not easily detected, hGH testing research for Sidney games, etc.

Doping and prevention of doping: international cooperation, by H. H. Hoppeler, et al. CLINICAL JOURNAL OF SPORT MEDICINE 5:79-81, 1995.
Editorial on testing and legal issues and education, suggesting a values-based approach; references.

Doping at the Olympics: clenbuterol, by J. White. PHYSICIAN AND SPORTS MEDICINE 20(10):19-20, October 1992.
Defines clenbuterol and explains briefly what it can do, illegal status in the U.S., and testing issues.

Doping control in sports medicine, by J. Segura. THERAPEUTIC DRUG MONITORING 18:471-476, 1996.
Explains what is involved, regulations, accreditation of labs, methods of analysis, what drugs are banned, and the potential of hair and saliva testing which is less invasive than testing urine or blood.

Doping in world sport, by R. Essick. SWIMMING WORLD AND JUNIOR SWIMMER 36:39-40, February 1995.
Position statement of U.S. swimming regarding testing in an effort to police its sport for cheaters is included and that FINA performed unannounced testing of Chinese in Hiroshima at Asian games.

The drug detectives, by R. Corelli and P. Gains. MACLEAN'S 109:28-29, July 22, 1996.
Good introduction to past and recent drug abuse in sports, testing procedures for the Atlanta Olympics, how athletes have attempted to beat the tests, and other testing changes.

Drug doping in senior Australian rules football: a survey for frequency, by K. J. Hardy, et al. BRITISH JOURNAL OF SPORTS MEDICINE 31:126-128, 1997.
Based on random, unannounced urine testing during 1990-1995, drug doping is not a problem (no positive results for AAS).

Drug testing project in international sports: dilemmas in an expanding regulatory regime, by J. B. Jacobs and B. Samuels. HASTINGS INTERNATIONAL AND COMPARATIVE LAW REVIEW 18:557-589, Spring 1995.
This is a very thorough examination of the drug-free international sport goal, challenges in terms of out-of-competition testing, technology of avoiding getting caught, finances, procedures of collecting urine samples, political problems, sanctions, and much more.

Drug use and control in sports [editorial], by M. G. Di Pasquale. DRUGS IN SPORTS 1(2):2-3, 1992.
Commentary on drug testing with recommendations.

Drugs in sport-chains of custody, by E. Grayson. NEW LAW JOURNAL 145:44+, January 20, 1995.
Comments on the lack of faith in drug testing procedures and specifically in the Diane Modahl case; Modahl contends the test was a false positive and a miscarriage of justice in Lisbon. Suggests IOC testing labs have a conflict of interest.

Drugs in sport: justifying paternalism on the grounds of harm, by S. Olivier. AMERICAN JOURNAL OF SPORTS MEDICINE 24:S43-S45, 1996.
Commentary/editorial/opinion expressed and explained concerning performance-enhancing substances, banning of a variety of ergogenic aids, and justifying that limitation in sport.

Drugs in sports, by D. MacAuley. BRITISH MEDICAL JOURNAL 313(7051):211-215, July 27, 1996.

This is an overview article on banned drugs, blood doping, testing results from London, testing procedures, and selected references.

East Germany: science in the disservice of the state, by S. Dickman. SCIENCE 254:26-27, October 4, 1991.

Previously secret East German documents uncovered by West German molecular biologist proves state-sponsored research to perfect steroid hormone drugs for athletes.

Effect of competition stress on tests used to assess testosterone administration in athletes, by C. Y. Guezennec, et al. INTERNATIONAL JOURNAL OF SPORTS MEDICINE 16:368-372, 1995.

Psychological stress does increase the production of steroid hormones, but does not influence the excretion of metabolites used to detect drug use.

Finding the most reliable dope on doping, by A. A. Skolnick. JAMA 275(5):349-350, February 7, 1995.

Brief factual information about drug testing for all athletes, including hot-lines for questions regarding banned substances by the IOC, NCAA; warns that similar sounding substances may not be the same and that OTC medications can contain illegal substances and beware of health food supplements/herbal.

Flora and furor, by L. Montville. SPORTS ILLUSTRATED 81:40-42, September 19, 1994.

The Chinese women's swim team has been extremely successful, but most suspect that they are on performance-enhancing drugs.

Forensic and technical aspects of drug testing in athletics, by R. H. B. Sample and J. C. Baenziger. SPORTS MEDICINE, TRAINING AND REHABILITATION 4: 257-274, 1993, reprinted from COMMENTS ON TOXICOLOGY 4:185-211, 1992.

Authors discuss in detail the collection procedures, rationale, analytical techniques, accreditation process, specific banned classes, side effects and health risks. An addendum notes some changes since first published, i.e. anabolic steroid class expanded to include clenbuterol and other ß-agonists, etc. This is a very readable article on a somewhat technical topic of doping control.

Forensic issues arising from the use of anabolic steroids, by C. C. Kleinman. PSYCHIATRIC ANNALS 20:219-221, 1990.

Two cases are summarized and compared from Maryland and Florida with different results. AAS-induced psychiatric illnesses resulted in criminal behavior and it must be decided whether to use insanity defense or whether to consider voluntary intoxification. Lack of premeditation depends on the state where tried.

Gas chromatographic/election impact mass spectrometric selective confirmatory analysis of clenbuterol in human and bovine urine, by A. Polettini, et al. BIO-LOGICAL MASS SPECTROMETRY 22:457-461, 1993.

Technical article on how to test for clenbuterol in human and bovine urine, horse racing was interested in stimulatory activity on respiration, but it was banned in 1985. Athletes interested in "anabolizing" effect, but IOC lists as a stimulant; screening method successfully used during Barcelona Olympic Games.

Illegal growth hormone marketing schemes alleged, by A. Tuffs. LANCET 344: 603, August 27, 1994.

Half-page report on Genentech, Inc., which engaged in illegal marketing of protropin which is a genetically engineered growth hormone for growth hormone deficiency; height screening of school children for purpose of promoting the drug is forbidden.

Injecting new life into an old defense: anabolic steroid-induced psychosis as a paradigm of involuntary intoxication, by M. J. Bidwill and D. L. Katz. UNIVERSITY OF MIAMI ENTERTAINMENT AND SPORTS LAW REVIEW 7:1-63, 1989.

Yet another thorough overview and discussion of the legal defense with extensive legal references and notes on steroid-induced psychosis and legal insanity, voluntary intoxication, involuntary intoxication, etc. is provided.

Inside the system: a conversation with an East German doping doctor, by S. Hartl. JOE WEIDER'S FLEX 15(6):204-208, August 1, 1997.

This is part five and the conclusion to the series (April-August 1997) on the East German doping practices from the perspective of an East German physician who is now in private general practice. He answers a series of questions about whether athletes were forced to take drugs, side effects, individual dosages, secrecy, growth hormone use, and possible long term effects. This doctor did not believe athletes were forced nor did he witness numerous side effects, but each club had its own doctors.

An insider's tale of doping, by P. Whitten. SWIMMING WORLD AND JUNIOR SWIMMER 35:38, June 1994.

Further discussion about the Chinese doping situation and comparison with East Germany in 1988 and 1989 when women swimmers tested positive for masking agents.

International cooperation in analytical chemistry: experiences of antidoping control at the XI Pan American Games, by J. Segura, et al. CLINICAL CHEMISTRY 39:836-845, 1993.

Very technical article about specific testing methods and testing results about specific drugs. Trend toward a decrease in the use of prohibited substances. Anti-asthmatic salbutamol mentioned as declared by athletes.

The intersection of law and policy: drug testing in sport, by A. Buti and S. Fridman. AUSTRALIAN JOURNAL OF PUBLIC ADMINISTRATION 53:489-507, 1994

This is a well written and very readable article that questions the wide acceptance of drug testing and the legality of testing athletes, i.e., privacy invasion, purpose, restraint of trade issue; warns that positive test results have been successfully challenged.

Jessica Foschi issue, by P. Whitten. SWIMMING WORLD AND JUNIOR SWIMMER 31(1):10-13, 1996.

Reports the decision of a review board to give 15-year-old Jessica Foschi, who tested positive for AAS, two years probation rather than suspension like the Chinese swimmers; much international criticism, but U.S. claims sabotage and Foschi passed lie detector test and questions the accuracy of the drug test.

Junk juice: counterfeit and designer steroids, by M. G. Di Pasquale. JOE WEIDER'S FLEX 13(10):143-148+, November 1, 1995.

Warns that designer steroids could be counterfeit and tells how to distinguish inert substances and other fakes and the real active drugs, i.e. check labeling, packet inserts, etc.; chemical and biological impurities can be dangerous.

The kids aren't alright, by S. Hartl. JOE WEIDER'S FLEX 15(4):139-143, June 1, 1997.
> This is the third in a five-part series (April-August 1997) on the East German doping system. Adolescents and children were given anabolic steroids and other drugs to enhance their athletic training and performance without parental consent. Women athletes were subjected to systematic doping with anabolic steroids despite side effects. Physicians would use tests to determine optimum dosages.

Law and athlete drug testing in Canada, by J. de Pencier. MARQUETTE SPORTS LAW JOURNAL 4:259-299, 1994.
> Excellent overview of Canadian law governing bodies and organizations and comparisons with Australian legislation; author feels that legal aspects and challenges are becoming the focus rather than doping control.

Legal regimes for the control of performance-enhancing drugs in sport, by H. Opie. ADELAIDE LAW REVIEW 12:332-355, 1990.
> Reviews the banned drugs, anti-doping rules in the Olympic Charter, definitions, specific cases, IAAF anti-doping rules, authority to test and rights of privacy, discipline.

Legalize and regulate: a prescription for reforming anabolic steroid legislation, by J. Burge. LOYOLA OF LOS ANGELES ENTERTAINMENT LAW JOURNAL 15:33-60, 1994.
> Reviews what steroids can do, sources of information, legislation, regulation, etc.; recommends legalization and regulation of AAS as prescription drugs; compares announced and random testing which can be very expensive.

Of MDs and muscles—lessons from two "retired steroid doctors," by D. L. Breo. JAMA 263:1697+, March 23-30, 1990.
> Summarizes some of the Dublin Inquiry testimony in Canada; Ben Johnson's doctor, Astaphan, and Kerr, AAS expert physician from early 1980s in California, are described as two steroid doctors, but Kerr now speaks out against AAS.

On your mark, get set, stop! Drug-testing appeals in the International Amateur Athletic Federation, by H. J. Hatch. LOYOLA OF LOS ANGELES INTERNATIONAL AND COMPARATIVE LAW JOURNAL 16:537-568, 1994.
> Suggests independent arbitration to dispute IAAF finding; international sport law is technical and complicated; discussion of the Butch Reynolds Supreme Court case vs. IAAF.

Over the edge, by M. Bamberger and D. Yaeger. SPORTS ILLUSTRATED 86(15): 60-67, April 14, 1997.
> This is an overview and commentary on testing issues at the Atlanta Olympics. Authors report on designer steroids which are chemically altered to tailor to athlete's needs and make them more difficult to detect, human growth hormone, EPO, insulin growth factor-1, and bromantan.

Parade's guide to better fitness, by M. O'Shea. PARADE MAGAZINE October 18, 1992, p. 18.
> Q&A format on the use of steroids and FBI efforts, how to spot steroid use, and sources of information.

Performance-enhancing drugs, fair competition, and Olympic sport, by D. H. Catlin and T. H. Murray. JAMA 276:231-237, July 17, 1996.
Very thorough discussion of what classes are banned, testing at Olympics, what happened with positive test, procedures, and much more.

Pharmacoepidemiology of the drugs used in sports as doping agents, by G. Benzi. PHARMACOLOGICAL RESEARCH 29:13-26, 1994.
Doping definition, testing laboratories and lack of them in most countries, commentary about not enough testing, extensive graphs, IOC banned list of drugs (always dated), lack of scientific evidence, and misinformation that prevails, etc. are all covered.

Playing by the rules? A legal analysis of the United States Olympic Committee—Soviet Olympic Committee doping control agreement, by M. T. Wolff. STANFORD JOURNAL OF INTERNATIONAL LAW 25:611-646, 1989.
Examines the USOC and Soviet OC doping control agreement to work together to eliminate athletes' blood-doping and use of ergogenic drugs.

Potential use of ketoconazole in a dynamic endocrine test to differentiate between biological outliers and testosterone use by athletes, by A. T. Kicman. CLINICAL CHEMISTRY 39:1798-1802, 1993.
Technical article about a method for detecting the administration of androgens such as testosterone by ratio of testosterone to epitestosterone (T/E) in urine as evidence of offense. "Investigations are currently underway to develop the ketocanazole test."

Proscription drugs: state-sponsored doping theory loses credit, by M. Forney. FAR EASTERN ECONOMIC REVIEW 159:56-57, July 4, 1996.
This is a brief report on the doping scandal involving China's runners and swimmers and a single Swede drug tester who began in 1994 to test Chinese athletes in preparation for the Atlanta Olympics. Some comparisons between East Germany and China are made, but no East German coaches had been discovered in China. This is part of a larger issue devoted to Chinese athletes and their desire for financial reward.

Random testing of professional athletes, by A. C. Page. WILLIAM AND MARY LAW REVIEW 33:155-160, 1991.
Discusses the Substance Abuse Testing Act of 1991 and argues that athletes' privacy interests are basic and that random testing of professional athletes does not solve the nation's substance abuse problems.

Recent developments in Canadian sports law, by J. Barnes. OTTAWA LAW REVIEW 23:623-706, 1991.
Thorough overview of Canadian federal programs and policies, doping control, legal and constitutional aspects, privacy right, Ben Johnson and the Dublin Report, commercialism of professional sport, collective bargaining and contractual issues.

Regulation of anabolic steroids, by J. S. Koeze. SCHOOL LAW BULLETIN 21:8-10, Summer 1990.
Brief overview of regulations under federal and North Carolina laws.

Run of the pill (argument against anti-drug policies in sports), by E. Cashmore. NEW STATESMAN AND SOCIETY 7:22-23, November 11, 1994.
Argues against banning drugs in sports because it increases their attraction but does not make athletes safe or competition fair.

Screening for diuretics in urine and blood serum by capillary zone electrophoresis, by H. S. Jumppanen and M. L. Riekkola. JOURNAL OF CHROMATOGRAPHY 652:441-450, 1993.
Very technical article about CZE method for screening for diuretics, which are used by athletes for losing weight and masking the use of anabolic steroids; electropherograms and chromatograms illustrate.

Sentinel effect of drug testing for anabolic steroid abuse, by R. J. Fuentes, et al. JOURNAL OF LAW, MEDICINE AND ETHICS 22(3):224-230, Fall 1994.
Makes the case for year-round random drug testing as an effective deterrent and thus supports the banning of anabolic steroids in athletics.

Serum and urine hormonal profiles for detecting testosterone and anabolic steroid use [update], by M. G. Di Pasquale. DRUGS IN SPORTS 2(2-3):6-8, 1993.
Commentary and further explanation of the urinary testosterone/ epitestosterone ratio used to detect doping by athletes; other factors can affect the ratios and may even cause false positives.

A simulated growth hormone analysis, by M. Harris. JOURNAL OF CHEMICAL EDUCATION 73:735-737, 1996.
Drug testing for growth hormone can provide real world application of a simulated urine sample analysis for lysozyme.

Sports Illustrated gets an "F" on NFL drug testing article, by G. C Griffin. POSTGRADUATE MEDICINE 86:13-16, 1989.
Editorial about the critical article on NFL drug testing; author recommends more drug testing and especially random testing.

Sports Illustrated, the "war on drugs," and the Anabolic Steroid Control Act of 1990, by B. E. Denham. JOURNAL OF SPORT AND SOCIAL ISSUES 21(3): 260-273, August 1997.
Author reviews several major cover stories and other Sports Illustrated articles about the dangers of steroids and suggests that the popular magazine had some influence on the enacting of legislation to control steroids. Author also suggests a contradiction in that the public enjoys watching violent football and large lean bodybuilders and wrestlers, but wants to reduce the availability of steroids.

Steroids for endurance?, by M. C. Siff. FITNESS AND SPORTS REVIEW INTERNATIONAL 29:151-152, 1994.
Claims that Chinese athletes have been using anabolic steroids successfully in both strength and endurance sports and comments on testing inconsistencies; recommends that there be two competitors: drug-free and drug-assisted.

Steroids: wrestling with the issues, by E. L. Ham. TRIAL 29:36-42, 1993.
Summarizes several issues including the rage defense or "dumbbell" defense, "roid rage," Anabolic Steroid Control Act, "roid psych," regulation, testing and trafficking. Author recommends education about the harmful effects of steroids.

Stricter drug testing in sports and elsewhere, by G. C. Griffin. POSTGRADUATE MEDICINE 84:11-12+, 1988.
Editorial on drug testing issues of fairness and cost and more.

Swimming for her country's honor, by S. V. Lawrence. US NEWS AND WORLD REPORT 12/25/95, January 1, 1996, p. 100.

> One-page with illustration about Liu Limin training for the butterfly event after 11 Chinese athletes failed drug tests in 1994 at Asian Games; briefly describes the strict discipline and routine of Chinese swimmer.

Testing for drug abuse, by J. Honour. LANCET 348:41-43, July 6, 1996.

> Discusses the testing results of British athlete, Diane Modahl, using testosterone to epitestosterone ratio (40/1); Modahl won her appeal and is seeking damages; further discussion of testing issues and other drugs.

They shoot horses, don't they? Anabolic steroids and their challenge to law enforcement, by G. Stejskal. FBI LAW ENFORCEMENT BULLETIN August 1994, pp. 1-6.

> Reviews history of steroid abuse and black market operations of Equine which led to the indictment of several Canadian steroid suppliers; also discusses sources in Mexico and Europe; profile of steroid distributor.

Top Chinese swimmer banned, by P. Whitten. SWIMMING WORLD AND JUNIOR SWIMMER 35:22, April 1994.

> Reports that China's top female swimmer, Zhong Weiyue, failed a drug test at a World Cup meeting in Beijing and was banned by FINA from international competition for two years. The substance found was an anabolic steroid, the same substance found in another Chinese woman swimmer a year earlier.

Tougher drug tests for Centennial Olympic Games, by A. A. Skolnick. JAMA 275(5):348-349, February 7, 1995.

> Reports that the Atlanta Summer Olympics in 1996 was to have the most strict drug testing by the USOC; discusses in brief the doping mentality and the results of a study of high school football players from Portland, Oregon; reports new tests being studied to detect exogenous testosterone.

Uncertain gold: drug testing at the Olympics, by D. Noble. ANALYTICAL CHEMISTRY 67:319A-321A, May 1, 1995.

> Somewhat technical but good overview which predicts that blood testing will be used in the near future.

Under suspicion, by M. Bamberger. SPORTS ILLUSTRATED 86(15):72-80, April 14, 1997.

> This article reports on the Irish swimmer and gold medalist from the Atlanta Olympics, Michelle Smith, including an interview with her and her husband/trainer concerning the accusations of illegal drug use. The author presents her swimming championship results over the years leading up to the Olympics, observations which have cast suspicion on her training methods, pre-Olympics absence while she was either in the Netherlands, Eastern Europe or Moscow, scandalous Irish coaches who have either been arrested, fled Ireland, or convicted of murder, and strained relationship with her parents. Smith has a book, Gold: A Triple Champion's Story, which is not available in the U.S. Bamberger speculates about why Smith has received such little post-Olympic acclaim.

U.S. Court exonerates track star (Harry Reynolds Jr., accused of steroid use by International Amateur Athletic Federation), by Z. Hale. NATIONAL LAW JOURNAL 15:10, January 25, 1993.
Reports that the federal judge ruled in favor of Reynolds, saying that the drug tests were flawed and inadequate; IAAF refused to recognize the court's jurisdiction.

Why are people saying all those nasty things about a nice Irish girl like Michelle Smith?, by P. Whitten. SWIMMING WORLD AND JUNIOR SWIMMER 38(1): 31-32, 1997.
Reviews reasons why athletes doubt that Michelle Smith could improve speed so dramatically at age 26 after years of hard work, but mediocre international results; EPO suspected because of success in endurance event and coaching by husband who was banned due to positive AAS test.

This subsection of testing legal issues gathers articles on the Fourth and Fourteenth Amendments to the U.S. Constitution, issues of privacy, school searches, reasonable suspicion as opposed to random suspicionless drug testing of college and younger athletes, college/university drug testing policies and procedures, and especially articles on Vernonia v. Acton and public school student athletes.

Acton and its impact on random, suspicionless drug testing of student athletes, by M. Little. UNIVERSITY OF LOUISVILLE JOURNAL OF FAMILY LAW 35(2):379-392, Spring 1996.
Author concurs with the Vernonia v. Acton Supreme Court decision and says that it was unfortunate that the policy was limited to student-athletes. Author reviews related cases, fairness of Acton, suggestions for schools.

Athletics, drug testing and the right to privacy: a question of balance, by S. O. Ludd. HOWARD LAW JOURNAL 34(4):599-632, 1991.
Author reviews constitutional theories and historical interpretations as applied to mandatory random drug testing in athletics, compares and contrasts professional, college and high school and essentially predicts the expansion of mandatory drug testing in American athletics. He does not see athletics in the same league with customs officials or public transportation etc. that may effect public safety and insists that reasonable suspicion of drug use be required to justify urine testing of athletes. Author recommends educationally based rehabilitation.

The boiling frog: privacy rights hang in the balance in Vernonia School District v. Acton, by K. J. Berets. WISCONSIN LAW REVIEW pp. 1101-1120, 1996.
Author states that ". . . Vernonia exposes millions of public elementary and high school students to school-mandated random drug testing" and urges the Supreme Court to reconsider its interpretation of the appropriate standard for a urinalysis search of student athletes. The intrusion may be minimal on one athlete, but added together amounts to a large invasion. Massive searches on school children becomes a general warrant.

California-NCAA drug testing invades privacy. SPORTS AND THE COURTS 13:5-7, 1992.
Summarizes particular case, Hill vs. NCAA, 1990, in which two Stanford

students complained that NCAA drug testing violated their right to privacy under the California Constitution; NCAA may not require student-athletes to waive constitutional rights in order to participate in intercollegiate athletics.

A casualty of the "War on Drugs": mandatory, suspicionless drug testing of student athletes in Vernonia School District 47J v. Acton, by M. Hallam. NORTH CAROLINA LAW REVIEW 74(3):833-862, March 1996.
Reviews the facts of Vernonia v. Acton, outcomes in lower courts, history of administrative searches under the Fourth Amendment, recent judicial treatment of school searches and drug testing, and more. Author concludes that school-wide drug testing, especially voluntary testing programs, are very possible.

Chemical warfare: battling steroids in athletics, by J. Thurston. MARQUETTE SPORTS LAW JOURNAL 1(1):93-148, 1990.
Author begins with an overview of the use of anabolic steroids by athletes, brief history, physical effects, black market, testing methods, etc. and then continues with a discussion and explanation of the constitutionality of drug testing, comparing professional, collegiate, and high school and making distinctions between anabolic steroid use and street or social drugs. He defines legal terms and interpretations and provides examples of court cases as well as extensive and clearly articulated footnotes. Sample drug testing consent form statements are provided. Author supports random unannounced steroid testing for athletes. He also notes that athletes have diminished expectations of privacy due to physical exams, communal showers and dressing rooms, and the voluntary nature of participation.

The coarsening of our national manner: the Supreme Court's failure to protect privacy interest of school children—Vernonia School District 47J v. Acton, by G. M. Dery, III. SUFFOLK UNIVERSITY LAW REVIEW 29(3):693-735, Fall 1995.
Author affirms that students should not have to waive their privacy rights merely because they must attend school, endure physical exams, or use and share the locker room and bathrooms. Author points out that Vernonia officials observed a drug problem at the high school and instituted a policy that included grade school. Individualized suspicion should be required and teachers/coaches should determine probable cause for suspicion of drug use.

College and university policies on substance abuse and drug testing. ACADEME 78:17-23, 1992.
Summarizes the report and response of the Association's Committee A on Academic Freedom and Tenure, February 1992, which warns that anti-drug and alcohol policies and drug-testing threaten academic norms and individual privacy interests. It would be better to direct efforts toward education and rehabilitation rather than punitive actions.

College athletes and drug testing: attitude and behaviors by gender and sport, by D. Schneider and J. Morris. JOURNAL OF ATHLETIC TRAINING 28:146-150, 1993.
Survey of attitudes of varsity athletes concerning mandatory drug testing and education and comparison of different sports and gender. Players felt coaches and trainers should also be tested, but basically expressed indifference.

Colorado-University's drug-testing program fails constitutional challenge. SPORTS AND THE COURTS 14:7-8, 1993.

> Summarizes the case, Derdeyn vs. University of Colorado, 1991, in which the Appellate Court agreed only on "reasonable suspicion," but urinalysis was considered a search under the constitution.

Compensating behavior and the drug testing of high school athletes, by R. Taylor. CATO JOURNAL 16(3):351-364, Winter 1997.

> Theoretical analysis with formulas that suggests that drug testing may not have the desired result of reducing drug use by student athletes; drug use may actually increase among ex-athletes who have been discouraged from participation in sports. Author recommends careful studies during implementation of random drug testing programs.

Computers, urinals, and the Fourth Amendment: confessions of a patron saint, by W. R. LaFave. MICHIGAN LAW REVIEW 94:2553-2589, 1996.

> After a wordy and long introduction, specific cases, including Vernonia vs. Acton, are discussed and compared; extensive notes. Author, an expert on the Fourth Amendment and search and seizure, warns that the Acton case decision by the Supreme Court has further eroded the Fourth Amendment protections. He also warns that other suspicionless search programs will be upheld.

The Constitution expelled: what remains of students' Fourth Amendment rights?, by D. Jackson. ARIZONA STATE LAW JOURNAL 28:673-698, 1996.

> Author provides a history of student rights, analyzes Vernonia v. Acton, and examines the possible consequences of the departure from previous Supreme Court decisions regarding suspicionless drug testing and searches in school. The Constitution does not apply with equal force to students. Warrants and probable cause requirements are not necessary if the state can demonstrate a special need. Author notes that Vernonia teachers might have been better able to maintain discipline had they been allowed to recommend drug testing based on individualized suspicion. Author also predicts that random, suspicionless, school-wide testing may be allowed and that this will have a negative impact on student attitudes about government.

Constitutional law—Fourth Amendment—another slice of the right to privacy pie: do public school children maintain any Fourth Amendment rights after Vernonia Sch. Dist. 47J v. Acton, 115 S. Ct. 2386 (1995):, by C. L. Mears. SOUTH TEXAS LAW REVIEW 37:591-607, 1996.

> Author states that the Supreme Court's majority decision in Vernonia v. Acton opens the door for random, suspicionless drug testing of all public school students. The Court's comparison of monitored urinalysis to public restroom situations is incorrect. The distinction between athletes and general student population who are required to take physical education classes is very minimal. Author concludes that the Court's decision has equated the public school child's status to that of a prisoner. The author asks when the "compelling" state interest will be overridden so as to maintain some rights to privacy in school bathrooms and locker rooms, purses and wallets, etc.

Constitutional law—search and seizure—random, warrantless, and suspicionless searches of student athletes through urinalysis drug testing by public school officials does not violate Fourth Amendment, by R. L. Diehl. SETON HALL LAW REVIEW 27(1):230-259, Winter 1997.

Author reviews the Vernonia v. Acton case and other related drug testing cases, etc. and concludes that the Supreme Court's decision allows school officials to overstep their authority. Author supports the dissenting minority viewpoint that a suspicion-based program would achieve Vernonia's goal without denying innocent students their privacy rights.

Constitutional law—testing the Fourth Amendment: random, suspicionless urinalysis drug-testing of student-athletes is unconstitutional search—University of Colorado v. Derdeyn 863 P.2d 929 (Colo. 1993), by S. B. Blair. SUFFOLK UNIVERSITY LAW REVIEW 28:217-227, 1994.
Notes are longer and more detailed than commentary, but author says that educational institutions may have to rethink drug-testing of student athletes.

Constitutionality of drug testing of college-athletes: a Brandeis brief for a narrowly-intrusive approach, by J. T. Ranney. JOURNAL OF COLLEGE AND UNIVERSITY LAW 16(3):397-424, Winter 1990.
Explains the balancing of reasonable suspicion against need to intrude but insure privacy in specimen collection process, giving University of Montana model example.

Constitutionality of random drug testing of student athletes make the cut . . . but will the athletes?, by T. L. Arnold. JOURNAL OF LAW AND EDUCATION 25:190-198, 1996.
Author agrees with the Supreme Court majority that policy reasonable and not intrusive in the Vernonia School District vs. Acton, but did not include testing for steroids or alcohol.

Deciding whether to test student athletes for drug use, by C. D. Feinstein. INTERFACES 20:80-87, 1990.
Based on the author's decision-making model, the athletic governing board of Santa Clara University concluded that the incidence of drug use was so low and cost of false accusation so high that drug-testing was not correct; probability formulas and decision tree model included.

Do public school athletes shed their constitutional rights at the locker room door? The Supreme Court upholds random urinalysis drug testing of public school athletes: Vernonia vs. Acton, by L. Crossett. TEXAS TECH LAW REVIEW 27:327-350, 1996.
Reviews the Supreme Court decision regarding drug testing of student athletes in Oregon and asks some thought-provoking questions about what the decision means for Fourth Amendment safeguards.

Drug test passes court test, by P. A. Zirkel. PHI DELTA KAPPAN 77(2):187-188, 1995.
Another overview of the Supreme Court case (Vernonia vs. Acton) with some background, specific procedures outlined and comparison of majority and dissenting viewpoints.

Drug testing and the college athlete, by K. S. Covell and A. Gibbs. CREIGHTON LAW REVIEW 23:1-18, 1989-1990.
Describes programs for college student athletes, policy arguments in favor of and against drug testing and legal decisions, i.e. Stanford athletes refused to submit to mandatory drug testing, and right to privacy protection with state constitutions but not federal courts.

Drug testing and the evolution of Federal and State regulation of intercollegiate athletics: a chill wind blows, by W. L. Schaller. JOURNAL OF COLLEGE AND UNIVERSITY LAW 18:131-159, Fall 1991.

Reviews employment testing, Tarkanian case, NCAA; suggests rapid-eye exam useless; warns that drug testing risks exposure of those involved in illicit drug use in intercollegiate athletics; and recommends that universities use reasonable suspicion or probable cause rather than random testing.

Drug testing and the student-athlete: meeting the constitutional challenge, by C. F. Knapp. IOWA LAW REVIEW 76:107-138, 1990.

This is an excellent, readable legal review of the constitutionality of student-athlete drug testing, statistics on drug programs, privacy, equal protection, due process, etc.; states that drug testing under direct observation too invasive and may prove unconstitutional even though the athlete may have diminished expectations of privacy; extremely well referenced.

Drug testing, collective suspicion, and a Fourth Amendment out of balance [a reply to Professor Howard], by D. J. Gottlieb. KANSAS JOURNAL OF LAW AND PUBLIC POLICY 6:27-38, Winter 1997.

This author disagrees with Howard's support of the Supreme Court majority opinion in the Vernonia/Acton case and follows Howard's article in the same issue with a critical evaluation of constitutional interpretation, i.e. individualized suspicion should be required for a search to be reasonable as expressed by the minority opinion. Author also points out, as others have, that there was little evidence of a drug epidemic and that Vernonia did not test for alcohol or steroids.

Drug testing college athletes: NCAA does thy cup runneth over?, by S. F. Brock, et al. WEST VIRGINIA LAW REVIEW 97:53-114, 1994.

Excellent review of several college and to a lesser extent high school decisions concerning drug testing of amateur athletes. Thoroughly discusses the challenges to several university sponsored programs (Stanford, Colorado, Washington, Northwestern) and the NCAA's program on state constitutional levels. Considers and discusses the constitutionality of drug testing athletes and the notion of diminished expectations of privacy due to communal undressing and showering, but recommends alternatives to monitored urination. Drug use must also be documented to establish the need for testing and the NCAA should narrow its list of banned drugs to performance-enhancing (AAS. . .) and those that would be considered a health threat.

Drug testing: college jocks score win. ABA JOURNAL 80:77-78, 1994.

Brief news article reports that Colorado Supreme Court held that forcing intercollegiate athletes at University of Colorado to consent to random urine testing violates Fourth Amendment, i.e., the University's drug screening program was an unreasonable search/seizure that violated the students' privacy.

Drug testing high school and junior high school students after Vernonia School District 47J v. Acton: proposed guidelines for school districts, by A. P. Massmann. VALPARAISO UNIVERSITY LAW REVIEW 31(2):721-785, Spring 1997.

Author reviews briefly some of the lawsuits filed to challenge mandatory student testing, provides an overview of the Fourth Amendment, i.e. what constitutes a search, reasonableness and warrants, exceptions, balancing test, etc. This is a very thorough review which also proposes guidelines for school districts, suggesting that there be no observed urination, but rather that the male or female student be in an enclosed stall, that testing be voluntary rather than mandatory, that there should be an appeals process, and more. Author also reasons that a blanket program requiring all students to submit to random, suspicionless drug testing would not pass the Fourth Amendment reasonable test because just attending public school should not diminish expectations of privacy. However, other student groups besides athletes could be tested, but the author recommends guidelines be established and followed.

Drug testing high school athletes and the Fourth Amendment, by E. C. Bjorklun. EDUCATION LAW REPORTER 83:913-925, 1993.
The author begins with some review of steroid use statistics as well as alcohol and illicit drugs, drug testing and the Fourth Amendment, drug testing programs in several states, legal challenges, etc. and then reviews the legality of drug testing programs before the Supreme Court decision concerning the Vernonia School District. Author finally focuses in on what testing would be legal: aimed at a specific group (athletes), voluntary participation, random selection for testing, limited use of results and limited penalties.

Drug testing in intercollegiate Athletics-Hill v. National Collegiate Athletic Association, 26 Cal. Rpt. 2d 834 (Cal. 1994), by W. MacKnight. SETON HALL JOURNAL OF SPORT LAW 5:529-551, 1995.
Two athletes challenged the NCAA drug testing program based on privacy rights in the California State Constitution, but NCAA drug testing was upheld because the Hill majority decided that the NCAA as a private actor had a legitimate interest in preventing drug related sports injuries and this outweighed the privacy expectations of the student athletes. Intercollegiate athletics is highly regulated, students have advanced warning of testing, and must consent to participate. Author warns that many state constitutions may not allow a privacy action against the NCAA.

Drug testing of college athletes, by R. R. Albrecht, et al. SPORTS MEDICINE 14:349-352, 1992.
This is an editorial on the moral or ethical issues concerning right/wrong of athletes using ergogenic drugs, fair competition, rationale for testing, informed consent, confidentiality, expense of testing, and further discussion of NCAA testing and why.

—, by T. A. Leeson. JOURNAL OF COLLEGE AND UNIVERSITY LAW 16(2): 325-341, Fall 1989.
Suggests removing the monitoring of urination—take other precautions—but close door to stall for both NCAA and educational institutions; drug education strongly promoted as well as drug usage survey, counseling and rehabilitation.

Drug testing of high school student athletes after Vernonia, by A. T. Pittman and M. R. Slough. EDUCATION LAW REPORTER 104:162-174, December 4, 1995.
Author reviews statistics of drug abuse by athletes, including anabolic steroid use, drug testing and Fourth Amendment, state interest, facts about Vernonia v. Acton, including the change from mandatory to voluntary drug testing, and specific characteristics that are important for school districts. Steroids were not tested for because of the high cost. Author emphasizes that programs not be punitive.

Drug testing of student-athletes: another weapon in the war against drugs, by C. J. Russo and T. E. Morse. SCHOOL BUSINESS AFFAIRS 61:60-62, December 1, 1995.

> Case study discussion of Vernonia vs. Acton concerning the drug testing of a seventh grade male would-be football player; supports the decision to uphold the random testing.

Drug testing of student athletes in Vernonia School District v. Acton: Orwell's 1984 becomes Vernonia's reality in 1995, by S. Osheroff. LOYOLA OF LOS ANGELES ENTERTAINMENT LAW JOURNAL 16(2):513-540, Fall 1995.

> Author very succinctly reviews the case and related cases and concludes that the Vernonia drug testing policy should have been found to be unconstitutional because it was based on random testing without suspicion when it was clear that certain drug using students and/or those with disciplinary problems had been recognized. Acton's privacy rights and those of other innocent school children are damaged. Vernonia also did not test for the most popular drug, alcohol, nor for steroids, most likely to be misused by student-athletes to enhance performance.

Drug testing of student athletes: a policy concern, by D. Louria. NEW JERSEY MEDICINE 93:41-44, May 1996.

> Reviews the recent Supreme Court decision (Vernonia vs. Acton) to uphold suspicionless and random drug testing of student athletes and warns of decreasing privacy, false positive result, mislabeling, less than careful analysis. Makes some suggestions for medical educators.

Drug testing of student athletes: some contrast and tort implications, by L. Pernell. DENVER UNIVERSITY LAW REVIEW 67:279-300, 1990.

> Includes sample consent to testing and discussion of enforceability of consent as a matter of contract law. Duress/undue influence/unconscionability, these common law doctrines guard confidentiality and greater freedom of choice.

Drug testing of students in public schools: implications of Vernonia School District v. Acton for other types of school-related drug searches, by J. A. Stefkovich and G. M. O'Brien. EDUCATION LAW REPORTER 113:521-538, 1996.

> This commentary focuses on the unresolved issues and implications of Vernonia v. Acton, i.e., males have lesser expectations of privacy than females and thus can be observed providing urine sample; what constitutes a drug problem and thus how to document the severity of the need for drug testing; what about state requirements to report illegal drug use to law enforcement; could testing be extended to extracurricular activity involvement; references and notes.

Drug testing: proving your clean, by K. M. Kowalski. CURRENT HEALTH 2 23(3): 19-21, 1996.

> Reviews briefly the Vernonia vs. Acton case and explains testing procedures and methods. Mentions that drug-testing is done in the workplace and what happens if you test positive or fail the drug test. (Editors note: "Your" was the word used in title rather than you are or you're??!! as appeared in full-text database.)

Drugs and high school athletes, by L. Schnirring. PHYSICIAN AND SPORTS MEDICINE 23:25-26, 1995.

> Brief reaction and update to the Vernonia/Acton decision, reporting that school districts are unlikely to adopt similar policies of testing all student-athletes because the cost of testing is enormous. Peer counseling is mentioned as more effective than drug screening.

Drugs vs. Privacy: the new game in sports, by C. A. Palmer. MARQUETTE
SPORTS LAW JOURNAL 2:175-209, 1992.
"This article considers drug testing from the perspective of the high
school administrator who desires to adopt such a program." The author
reasons that a history of steroid abuse in high school supports drug testing of high school athletes. He also spells out regulations that should be
developed as well as sanctions for violation that will warn athletes and allow for expectations of privacy.

An evenhanded approach to diminishing student privacy rights under the Fourth
Amendment: Vernonia School District v. Acton, by M. A. Stanislawczyk.
CATHOLIC UNIVERSITY LAW REVIEW 45:1041-1099, 1996.
Author proposes a different test for balancing or weighing individual privacy and a compelling state interest. He concludes that the Ver-
nonia/Acton decision continues to reduce Fourth Amendment rights by
the elastic expansion of "compelling" and the minimization of student privacy expectations.

Expelling the Fourth Amendment from American schools: students' rights six
years after T.L.O., by J. M. Sanchez. JOURNAL OF LAW AND EDUCATION
21:381-413, 1992.
Although not specifically focused on drug testing, this article provides a
very detailed discussion of the T.L.O. case and school searches which
have been upheld because of T.L.O. for evidence of marijuana, alcohol,
cocaine, and other illegal drug use/possession/selling in schools.
Student's lockers and automobiles have been searched based on
information from anonymous phone calls, overheard conversations, or
student comments. Author says that these searches are invasions of
student's legitimate expectations of privacy.

The 4 R's of drug testing in public schools: random is reasonable and rights are
reduced, by J. J. Bursch. MINNESOTA LAW REVIEW 80:1221-1254, 1996.
This article discusses the federal trend to reduce public school students'
constitutional rights and Fourth Amendment protection, analyzes why,
proposes a random drug testing program for all public school students,
and thus agrees with the majority opinion of the Supreme Court in the
Vernonia v. Acton decision. Author reviews both pre-Acton and Acton
decisions and concludes that testing should extend beyond student
athletes with careful procedures, such as, no observation of student
providing sample, random selection, no criminal prosecution.

The Fourth Amendment and student drug testing policies: a split decision in the
federal courts, by T. A. DeMitchell. INTERNATIONAL JOURNAL OF EDU-
CATIONAL REFORM 4(3):362-368, 1995.
Author compares cases, reasonable as opposed to individualized
suspicion, student drug testing policies, random/blanket search,
conflicting decisions just before the Supreme Court's decision in late
June 1995 concerning Vernonia v. Acton.

Fourth Amendment protection of public school students: legal and psychological
inconsistencies, by S. Z. Ringel. MARYLAND JOURNAL OF
CONTEMPORARY LEGAL ISSUES 3(2):289-300, Spring 1992.
Though not specifically about athletes and drug testing, this author does
discuss privacy issues, diluted reasonable suspicion, student Fourth
Amendment protection, and thus encourages full privacy rights for
students.

Fourth & Fourteenth Amendments—search and seizure—public schools may constitutionally require students to submit to random testing in order to participate in varsity athletics, by J. M. Burke. SETON HALL LAW SCHOOL CONSTITUTIONAL LAW JOURNAL 7(1):223-241, Fall 1996.

> Author supports the Supreme Court's decision and argues that other decisions have made it clear that public school students have less expectations of privacy, i.e. more rules, less freedom, etc. and teachers must act in place of parents and protect athletes and reduce drug use.

Gone to pot: student athletes' Fourth Amendment rights after Vernonia School District 47J v. Acton, by C. E. Laszewski. SAINT LOUIS UNIVERSITY LAW JOURNAL 40(2):575-610, Spring 1996.

> Author thoroughly reviews the Vernonia case and other related cases on drug testing and warns that as governmental interest is weighed as more important than individual privacy, the law does not bode well for student athletes nor for public school students or public employees. Author challenges the Supreme Court to preserve the Fourth Amendment protections it does recognize.

Guilty until proven innocent: random urinalysis drug testing upheld in Vernonia School District 47J v. Acton, by J. S. Dressner. SPORTS LAWYERS JOURNAL 4(1):115-146, Spring 1996.

> Author analyzes the Vernonia v. Acton decision, comparing and contrasting earlier cases as well as the majority and minority opinions. Author states that the suspicion-based policy would be more effective in controlling drug use and unwanted behavior throughout the student body and least intrusive.

Hitting the mark: Vernonia School District v. Acton, by B. W. Martell. UNIVERSITY OF SAN FRANCISCO LAW REVIEW 31(1):223-256, Fall 1996.

> Author supports the Supreme Court decision and suggests instances of expansion, i.e. driver's education and physical education. Author does caution that positive drug test results are not to be used against the student in a law enforcement context, but the goal should be rehabilitative rather than punitive.

Indiana-court upholds high school drug-testing program. SPORTS AND THE COURTS 10:6-8, 1989.

> Summarizes the case, Schaill by Kross vs. Tippecanoe County School Corporation, which involved several high school athletes challenging the legality of the drug-testing policy; this was one of the first cases to deal with the educational sports setting and public policy and welfare versus individual rights.

Judicial activism works the Constitution out of shape—Acton and its atrophic effect on the Fourth Amendment rights of student athletes, by C. E. Samay. SETON HALL JOURNAL OF SPORT LAW 7(1):291-314, Winter 1997.

> Author strongly disagrees with the Vernonia v. Acton decision and makes some predictions for further expansion of public school drug testing and thus the further reduction of Fourth Amendment privacy rights that open the way for drug testing of college students without requiring evidence of drug use.

Leveling the playing field, by H. J. Reske. ABA JOURNAL 81:40, 1995.

> Briefly reviews the Supreme Court case, Vernonia School District vs. Acton, in which Oregon school district's drug testing program challenges the constitutional rights of the Fourth Amendment and raises the question of school children's individual privacy rights.

Mandatory drug testing of student athletes: a policy response to Vernonia School District 47J v. Acton, by T. A. DeMitchell and T. Carroll. JOURNAL OF SCHOOL LEADERSHIP 7:50-68, 1997.

This reports on a survey of randomly selected superintendents from five geographic regions of the U.S. to determine if they have enacted policy in response to Vernonia/Acton and if they believe drug testing will combat drug use. Majority were not planning on adopting similar drug testing policies.

Mass and intrusive searches of students in public schools, by J. A. Stefkovich. JOURNAL FOR A JUST AND CARING EDUCATION 2(3):229-241, July 1996.

Author reviews the reasonable suspicion standard as compared to the probable cause standard, explains and provides examples of mass searches of students in public schools, and comments that individualized suspicion has been sacrificed in order to wage war on drugs and violence. Author warns of a lack of clarity in the law concerning mass and intrusive searches, i.e. strip searches, drug testing, field trip luggage, locker, canine sniff, metal detector, etc. and school safety.

Message in a bottle: the United States Supreme Court decision in Vernonia School District 47J v. Acton, by D. E. Joubert. LOUISIANA LAW REVIEW 56:959-979, Summer 1996.

Author reviews Vernonia/Acton and related cases and concludes that if read literally, seems to be a sound decision. However, if Acton issued to apply to situations not covered by the facts of the case, then privacy rights protected by the Fourth Amendment could be restricted in ways not intended. The question left unanswered by Acton decision is whether drug testing could be extended to all student participants in extracurricular activities or even an entire student population.

Message in a bottle: Vernonia School District 47J v. Acton, by L. G. Peters. CREIGHTON LAW REVIEW 29(2):861-901, 1996.

Author reviews mass suspicionless search cases (border patrol, sobriety checkpoints, government employees and/or regulated industries) and concludes that Vernonia v. Acton did not involve the issue of public safety and thus did not justify mass random urinalysis of school children. No advance notice of testing was made, students were required to identify prescription medications, and monitors were coaches or teachers. There was also no evidence that students being tested at the grade school were drug users. Thus the Supreme Court decision in Vernonia v. Acton failed the reasonable test for suspicionless searches.

Mission impossible: a drug-free school environment, by F. Murray and M. Storm. SCHOLASTIC COACH 65(4):4-6, 1995.

This article describes the Lynchburg, Virginia drug-testing policy, methods and procedures, and specific costs.

The National Collegiate Athletic Association, random drug-testing and the applicability of the administrative search exception, by C. H. Thaler. HOFSTRA LAW REVIEW 17:641-588, 1989.

Discusses the Fourth Amendment "reasonableness" but that likely to survive constitutional challenge; extensive notes and references.

A national survey of drug testing policies for college athletics, by L. Fields, et al. MEDICINE AND SCIENCE IN SPORTS AND EXERCISE 26:682-686, 1994.

Using mailed questionnaires, authors surveyed colleges/universities regarding drug testing policies. Majority screen for drugs that hinder performance, i.e. cocaine/amphetamines not performance enhancing, i.e. steroids.

NCAA drug program: out of bounds but still in play, by J. M. Evans. JOURNAL OF LAW AND EDUCATION 19:161-191, 1990.
Good overview with some recommendations for change; covers procedures, federal/state constitutional limitations, search and seizure issues, etc.

The NCAA drug-testing and the California Constitution: has California expanded the right of privacy, by D. H. McBride. UNIVERSITY OF SAN FRANCISCO LAW REVIEW 23:253-290, 1989.
Lengthy and readable discussion of privacy and California case law, NCAA drug testing; decided in NCAA's favor as of 1994.

NCAA institutionally based drug testing: do our athletes know the rules of this game?, by R. R. Albrecht, et al. MEDICINE AND SCIENCE IN SPORTS AND EXERCISE 24:242-246, 1992.
College athletes were surveyed as to their awareness of drug testing programs and authors found misconceptions and ignorance; legal and informed consent are compared/contrasted.

NCAA state action: not present when regulating intercollegiate athletics—but does that include drug testing student athletes?, by A. Fecteau. SETON HALL JOURNAL OF SPORT LAW 5:291-312, 1995.
This is a legal discussion of the NCAA's authority, state action verses private actor, consideration of individual student-athletes, expectations of privacy; argues that the NCAA drug testing goes beyond college athletics to regulate the private lives of its athletes.

The NCAA's drug testing policies: walking a constitutional tightrope?, by W. T. Champion. NORTH DAKOTA LAW REVIEW 67:269-280, 1991.
The NCAA drug testing policies are unnecessary, expensive, humiliating, unconstitutional, illogical, counter-productive, intrusive rather than being based on reasonable suspicion and author recommends educational and impairment testing.

Nonconstitutional privacy based challenges to NCAA drug testing, by A. Saler. SPORTS LAWYERS JOURNAL 1:303-327, 1994.
Author thoroughly reviews the NCAA's drug testing procedures, discusses issues of consent and privacy and confidentiality, and concludes that a tort-based invasion of privacy claim will not be successful. He also states that legislatures are not likely to pass statutes limiting drug testing of college athletes. Student-Athlete Drug-Testing Consent form and Banned-Drug Classes are appended.

Public school drug testing: the impact of Acton, by I. M. Rosenberg. AMERICAN CRIMINAL LAW REVIEW 33:349-378, Winter 1996.
Thorough legal discussion (full of jargon) of the Vernonia vs. Acton Supreme Court case which upheld the public school district's right to conduct random drug testing of grade and high school students in order to determine eligibility to participate in interscholastic athletics. Author warns that the decision means less rights for children under the Fourth Amendment to the U.S. Constitution.

Random drug-testing high school student athletes in Vernonia School District 47J v. Acton: is the war on drugs a losing battle for the Fourth Amendment, by M. D. Mosser. WHITTIER LAW REVIEW 17:527-577, 1996.
Extremely thorough review of the Supreme Court case; author agrees with the decision but does express concern about confidentiality of test results. Also further warns that schools must pay close attention to what is disclosed and to whom. Reviews reasonableness of drug testing under the Fourth Amendment.

Random drug testing of high school athletes in New Jersey after Vernonia School District 47J v. Acton—will Acton make the cut?, by L. M. Bergamini. RUTGERS LAW REVIEW 49(2):551-593, Winter 1997.
Author thoroughly discusses the Vernonia v. Acton case and compares it to New Jersey decisions that have upheld greater privacy protection. Author says that since Vernonia, many high schools have instituted similar drug-testing policies. Author urges that state courts look carefully at state constitutions in order to afford students privacy protections that the Supreme Court has taken away. She summarizes that urinalysis is a search and not to be compared with communal undressing. So too monitored urination is offensive. New Jersey cases dealing with drug testing of public employees typically require individualized suspicion and thus this should apply to student athletes as well. She concludes that forcing students to comply with random drug testing as a condition of participation in interscholastic athletics forces them to prove their innocence and we should not sacrifice the freedoms and protections of students.

Random drug-testing of public school student athletes: a permissible search under the Fourth Amendment, by P. K. Madsen. BRIGHAM YOUNG UNIVERSITY JOURNAL OF LAW AND EDUCATION 97-111, Spring 1992.
Author reviews some statistics on drug use by school-age children, Schaill v. Tippecanoe, including the Tippecanoe student athlete drug education and testing program with sample consent form, Fourth Amendment, N.J. v. T.L.O., and then compares the cases. Author agrees with the decision to uphold drug testing in public schools, though this was before the Supreme Court's ruling in Vernonia v. Acton.

Random suspicionless drug testing of high school athletes, by S. E. Shutler. JOURNAL OF CRIMINAL LAW AND CRIMINOLOGY 86:1265-1303, 1996.
Lengthy legal discussion of the Vernonia vs. Acton case; author argues that the Supreme Court overstepped the boundaries of the Fourth Amendment in order to address America's drug problem. Vernonia provided very little evidence of athletes using drugs nor should they have diminished privacy.

Random urinalysis testing of student athletes—the "reasonable" resolution of a complex problem, by D. S. Swanson. SOUTHERN ILLINOIS UNIVERSITY LAW JOURNAL 21:651-673, Spring 1997.
Author concurs with the Supreme Court majority decision in Vernonia v. Acton that the student athlete drug testing policy did not violate the Fourth Amendment. Author explains the reasonableness test as it applies to school districts. She also discusses reactions by other school districts, some of which have decided not to implement random drug testing and others that are developing policies. Cost, confidentiality, intrusiveness, need for individualized suspicion, limitations, drug problem, etc. are concerns briefly considered.

Reforming the NCAA drug-testing program to withstand state constitutional scrutiny: an analysis and proposal, by T. P. Simon. UNIVERSITY OF MICHIGAN JOURNAL OF LAW REFORM 24:289-310, Fall 1990.
Reviews the NCAA drug-testing program, Fourth Amendment, year-round off-season training and out-of-competition testing, and recommends the NCAA limit to reasonable suspicion testing of athletes who show signs of AAS use.

The road not taken: judicial federalism, school, athletes, and drugs, by S. L. Wasby. ALBANY LAW REVIEW 59(5):1699-1707, 1996.
Discusses the decision made prior to the Supreme Court decision that upheld the Vernonia School District's drug testing policy; the decision of the U.S. Court of Appeals for the Ninth Circuit gave more weight to students' privacy than government interests based on interpretation of the Oregon Constitution.

Role of the Constitution in the drug testing of student athletes in the public school, by R. G. Deivert. JOURNAL OF ALCOHOL AND DRUG EDUCATION 36(2):32-41, Winter 1991.
Author reviews the history and reliability of drug testing, Fourth Amendment search and seizure issues, Fourteenth Amendment due process, and the constitutionality of drug testing long before the Vernonia v. Acton Supreme Court decision. Author reinforces that education and treatment are most important and minimal privacy intrusions.

Search and seizure-suspicionless drug testing—Seventh Circuit upholds drug testing of student athletes in the public schools—Schaill v. Tippecanoe County School Corp., 864 F.2d 1309 (7th Cir. 1988). HARVARD LAW REVIEW 103(2):591-597, 1989.
This is a short legal review of Schaill v. Tippecanoe with some comparisons to the National Treasury Employees Union v. Von Raab and Skinner v. Railway Labor Executives' Association cases which opened the door to widespread government drug testing in the workplace. Almost ten years before the Supreme Court decision in Vernonia v. Acton, random urine testing of public school athletes was upheld in Indiana. References a re also made to the New Jersey v. T.L.O. case which permitted the search of a student's purse on the basis of "reasonable suspicion."

Search and seizure: what your school's rights are, by J. A. Stefkovich and G. M. O'Brien. SCHOOL BUSINESS AFFAIRS 62:12-21, 1996.
Authors discuss school violence, cost of safety in terms of drug testing and searches for weapons and strip search cases, legal implications, NJ v. TLO and Vernonia v. Acton, and the Fourth Amendment. Authors warn that school officials cannot generalize court decisions to apply to different states or different situations. Annotated list of resources provided as well as references.

Searches in the absence of individualized suspicion: the case of Vernonia School District 47J v. Acton, by C. N. Floyd. ARKANSAS LAW REVIEW 50(2):335-362, 1997.
This is a thorough and very well explained review of Acton and previous related cases involving constitutional rights in school. Author disagrees with the majority view and concurs with the minority that drug testing should be based on individualized suspicion. Some school districts have now extended the testing to include all extracurricular activities not just athletic programs.

The significance of Oregon constitutional analysis in the administrative search context after Acton v. Vernonia School District 47J, by K. M. Woodworth. OREGON LAW REVIEW 75:609-631, Summer 1996.

The author reviews carefully the distinctive Oregon case law and compares and contrasts with the Supreme Court's Vernonia/Acton case decision and then the dilemmas to be faced by challenges to either state or federal courts. Oregon State Constitution is more protective than the U.S. Constitution.

Something terribly wrong here: Vernonia School District 47J v. Acton, 115 S. Ct. 2386 (1995), by S. L. Toussaint. NEBRASKA LAW REVIEW 75:151-180, 1996.

Author disagrees strongly with the majority opinion in Vernonia v. Acton and warns of a continuing trend to erode basic freedoms in order to deal with social problems. Also warns that other school districts will adopt drug testing policies. The Supreme Court's development of special needs exceptions under the Fourth Amendment has reduced individual protection. There has become an imbalance of power between the government and the individual and now even the elimination of probable cause as a requirement. Author discusses the proposal of a school district to test for steroids though only one to two athletes in a school might be using anabolic steroids. Steroids are likely to be used by only a limited group.

The status of student drug testing in the public schools after Schaill and Acton, by J. A. Stefkovich. ILLINOIS SCHOOL LAW QUARTERLY 15(2):58-71, 1995.

Author discusses drug testing and students' rights in the school setting, but before the Supreme Court decision regarding Vernonia v. Acton. Appropriate cases are cited and why different decisions reached in lower courts. Both Fourth and Fourteenth Amendment protections are reviewed. Author warns that drug testing may be sending the wrong message to school-age children in terms of democracy and constitutional rights. Schools should consider the least intrusive methods of education etc. before proposing a widespread drug testing program.

Student drug testing policies: the Supreme Court decides. Part Two, by T. A. DeMitchell. INTERNATIONAL JOURNAL OF EDUCATIONAL REFORM 4:488-495, 1995-1996.

Author reviews part one briefly, then the Vernonia/Acton decision, and concludes that students have the least measure of privacy protection. Author agrees with the dissenting minority that testing be based on suspicion of drug use, but also suggests a harsher penalty for positive result than missing the athletic season or counseling.

Students: caught in the crossfire of the war on drugs, by N. M. D'Alesandro. MARYLAND JOURNAL OF CONTEMPORARY LEGAL ISSUES 3(2): 233-261, Spring 1992.

Reviews drug testing cases before Vernonia v. Acton, application to the public schools, workplace, college and university, NCAA rules, high school cases, etc. Author urges school officials to resist implementing mandatory drug testing programs.

Students' Fourth Amendment rights and school safety, by J. A. Stefkovich and G. M. O'Brien. EDUCATION AND URBAN SOCIETY 29(2):149-161, February 1997.

> Authors review federal legislation, presidential directives, drug-free and safe school initiatives over the last twenty years; then they review Vernonia v. Acton and other selected cases. They also review policy implications for urban schools, i.e. advance notice, careful procedures to safeguard privacy and due process rights.

The Supreme Court's view of drug testing high school athletes, by L. J. Carpenter. STRATEGIES 9(5):13-16, February 1996.

> This brief article provides a very readable and succinct review of the Vernonia v. Acton Supreme Court decision of 6/26/95. Author explains very clearly and simply the legal doctrines of in loco parentis, Fourth and Fourteenth Amendments, privacy, and the constitutional review process.

Suspicionless drug testing and the Fourth Amendment, by K. C. Newsom. HARVARD JOURNAL OF LAW AND PUBLIC POLICY 19(1):209-216, Fall 1995.

> This author disagrees with the Supreme Court majority opinion in Vernonia vs. Acton and urges the application of standard of strict scrutiny to the Fourth Amendment to uphold privacy as a fundamental freedom.

Suspicionless drug testing of high school and college athletes after Acton: similarities and differences, by E. N. Miller. UNIVERSITY OF KANSAS LAW REVIEW 45(1);301-328, 1996.

> Author disagrees with the Supreme Court decision in Vernonia in that the school's drug testing policy should have been upheld as unconstitutional because its true goal was to stop drug abuse in the whole student body but only tested athletes. Also reviews the NCAA drug testing policy and that of state colleges and universities and determines those to be constitutional. Notes differences between college intercollegiate drug testing to ensure fair competition and h.s. and elementary policies that are meant to stop drug use of all students. Points out that monitored urination is much different than communal undressing for physical education or sport. Offers an alternative solution in that h.s. and elementary schools have suspicion-based testing of entire student body. This is a very good overview with readable and understandable explanations of the Fourth Amendment reasonableness factors and much more. Vernonia policy did not test for AAS and thus author questions whether seriously concerned with fair competition and/or health of athletes.

Tested positive: a Supreme Court decision shifts the standard for allowing drug testing, by G. M. Wong. ATHLETIC BUSINESS November 1995, pp. 10-14.

> Sports law report summarizes the facts of the U.S. Supreme Court decision (Vernonia vs. Acton) which upheld the right of public schools to randomly test student athletes for drugs.

Testing for drugs of abuse in children and adolescents, by R. Heyman, et al. PEDIATRICS 98(2):305-307, 1996.

> Detailed position statement of the American Academy of Pediatrics concerning the use of psychoactive drugs by children and adolescents and testing issues, especially in light of Supreme Court ruling . . . athletes should not be singled out for involuntary test.

To test or not to test: Article I, Section 7 and random drug-testing of Washington's public school student-athletes, by K. L. Helgeson. WASHINGTON LAW REVIEW 71:797-820, 1996.

This is a very thorough review of the Vernonia vs. Acton case in the context of Washington State Constitutional law as well as recommendations for student-athlete drug-testing. The author points out the need for individualized suspicion, reasonable belief, protection of private affairs (urination), and third party or independent non-school officials collection and testing. The author also suggests voluntary urinalysis, rather than coerced testing, handled off school grounds. Author concludes that Washington constitutional, common, and statutory law would not allow mandatory, random urinalysis as a condition for participation in interscholastic athletics.

Vernonia case comment: high school students lose their rights when they don their uniforms, by J. M. Ettman. NEW YORK LAW SCHOOL JOURNAL OF HUMAN RIGHTS 13(3):625-662, Spring 1997.

This author provides a thorough overview and then is very critical of the Supreme Court's decision to uphold random drug testing of student-athletes in an effort to control drug use and behavior problems. He reinforces the athlete's right to privacy and says that the Court's view of interscholastic athletics is very outdated, i.e. athletes do not usually shower at school, athletics is an integral part of education, activities do not pose a risk to the public, etc. Vernonia had no drug-related injuries. Vernonia's policy did not test for steroids which can pose a serious danger to young adolescents. The Court overlooked the requirement for probable cause/individualized suspicion. In future, the Court could declare constitutional the drug-testing of students before attending field trips. The author warns that the Court's reasoning makes drug-testing of all students possible.

Vernonia Sch. Dist. v. Acton: Now children must shed their constitutional rights at the schoolhouse gate, by J. A. Tappendorf. UNIVERSITY OF HAWAII LAW REVIEW 18(2):869-908, Summer/Fall 1996.

This author reviews the Vernonia case and other ones challenging the privacy rights of school children and then makes comparisons with cases decided in Hawaiian courts. She points out that Vernonia concerned itself with keeping student-athletes drug-free which has little to do with public safety. Also she reiterates that monitored urine testing is offensive and not a reasonable method to deter drug use by young school children.

Vernonia School District 47J v. Acton: the decimation of public school students' Fourth Amendment rights, by S. J. Poturalski. UNIVERSITY OF TOLEDO LAW REVIEW 27(2):505-543, Winter 1996.

Author reviews case law thoroughly regarding students' right to privacy and the Fourth Amendment and concludes that the government has seriously intruded on constitutional rights in the name of maintaining classroom discipline and public policy against illegal drug use. He says that the Supreme Court could have made a more persuasive argument in Vernonia v. Acton by relying on Schaill v. Tippecanoe . . . which cited the high visibility of drug testing of collegiate, Olympic and professional athletes and thus student-athletes' lesser privacy expectations.

63

Vernonia School District 47J v. Acton: defining the constitutional scope of random suspicionless drug testing in inter-scholastic athletics and beyond, by A. J. Barker. WIDENER JOURNAL OF PUBLIC LAW 5:445-501, 1996.
> Author provides a very thorough review of the background and history of the reasonableness standard, "special needs" exception to the warrant requirement, and the development of suspicionless drug testing in public schools. Author proposes some specific scenarios for the possible further expansion of random suspicionless drug testing of students who voluntarily participate in extracurricular activities or of all public school students because of a perceived national drug abuse problem. The balancing test provides little protection.

Vernonia School District 47J v. Acton: the demise of individualized suspicion in Fourth Amendment searches and seizures, by C. S. Hagge. TULSA LAW JOURNAL 31:559-583, 1995-1996.
> Author reviews the history of the Fourth Amendment, recent developments in terms of the balancing test, requirement of individualized suspicion, privacy interest, nature of intrusion and governmental concern, and points out distinctions between other cases and Vernonia/Acton, i.e. evidence involved situations in which suspicion was present and a suspicion-based policy would have been effective.

Vernonia School District 47J v. Acton: flushing the Fourth Amendment—student athletes' privacy interests go down the drain, by J. G. Padilla. DENVER UNIVERSITY LAW REVIEW 73(2):571-596, 1996.
> Author is very critical of the majority decision in Vernonia v. Acton and discusses the very different opinions that Justice Scalia has about the invasion of privacy rights for adults as opposed to children. Author emphasizes the difference between the criminal search (N.J. v. T.L.O.) and administrative search. Author summarizes that Acton continues to erode the fundamental constitutional requirement that searches satisfy the reasonableness test.

Vernonia School District 47J v. Acton: a further erosion of the Fourth Amendment, by J. L. Malin. BROOKLYN LAW REVIEW 62:469-518, 1996.
> This is a well-reasoned, readable and understandable review of the Vernonia case along with a proposal to use the two-prong measure of strict scrutiny with suspicionless searches and intermediate scrutiny with reasonable suspicion. Author argues that in evaluating school searches, the nature of the privacy interest and the search determine whether strict or intermediate scrutiny is applied. The least intrusive alternative must be applied when a suspicionless search is imposed, but in Vernonia, the drug test was highly intrusive.

Vernonia School District 47J v. Acton: the right response for drug testing of student athletes, by R. C. Howard, Jr. KANSAS JOURNAL OF LAW AND PUBLIC POLICY 6(2):17-26, Winter 1997.
> This author agreed with the Supreme Court decision because he saw the testing as no more than a physical examination. He compares mass urinalysis to eye exams required for state driver's license or the use of metal detectors at airports for all travelers.

Vernonia School District 47J v. Acton: a step toward upholding suspicionless dog sniff searches in public schools, by J. Bradfield. UNIVERSITY OF COLORADO LAW REVIEW 68:475-505, Spring 1997.
> Author reviews the constitutionality of dog sniff searches and then focuses on the public school setting, comparing cases that reached different conclusions. Author comments on whether dog sniffing of student

lockers and possibly the students themselves would be upheld based on the Vernonia/Acton decision.

Vernonia School District 47J v. Acton: suspicionless drug testing of student-athletes held reasonable under the Supreme Court's balancing test, by D. R. York. JOURNAL OF CONTEMPORARY LAW 22:281-292, 1996.
This is a relatively brief overview of the Vernonia/Acton case, with some background and analysis of student-athlete privacy expectations, urinalysis testing, governmental interest, and dissent.

Vernonia School District 47J v. Acton: an unacceptable intrusion into student privacy, by T. Kirkby. THOMAS M. COOLEY LAW REVIEW 13(2):643-675, May 1996.
Author concludes that the Vernonia School District's drug testing policy was unreasonable. Vernonia School District did not have any actual evidence of drug use among student athletes. It also did not test for the two potentially most dangerous drugs: alcohol and steroids. Vernonia did not mention trying to educate teachers in how to recognize drug use among students, but blamed drug use for classroom disruption. Being monitored by known teachers/coaches can be traumatic for adolescents and thus very intrusive. Author also uniquely points out that student-athletes may have to give up educational and career opportunities in order to preserve their constitutional right to be free from unreasonable search in terms of urine testing. Interscholastic sports are often a way to obtain college scholarships and future coaching or recreational positions. Thus the Vernonia policy was an invasion on student privacy and it did not achieve the goal of protecting student-athletes from drug-related injuries.

Vernonia v. Acton: should schools conduct random drug test on student athletes?, by J. P. Mahon. NASSP BULLETIN 79:52-55, 1995.
Reviews briefly the Supreme Court case, reasons for the decision, and impact on schools.

Who will speak for the teachers? Precedent prevails in Vernonia School District 47J v. Acton, by A. G. Buzbee. HOUSTON LAW REVIEW 33:1229-1265, 1996.
This legal note makes a convincing argument for extending the suspicionless testing of all school children not just student athletes. He states that the nature of the child's relationship with the state (public school) reduces the expectation of privacy and that drug testing of all school children empowers teachers and administrators to maintain order. Buzbee argues that there is no difference between the student athlete and nonathlete. He maintains that drug-free schools are as important as enforcement of the Nation's laws against drug importation and preventing illegal aliens from entering the country. Author reviews other cases involving the reasonable search under the Fourth Amendment.

Will the real Fourth Amendment please stand up?, by D. A. Dripps. TRIAL 31(11):80-81, 1995.
Author says that the Acton decision only serves to confuse and contradict other decisions based on the Fourth Amendment because no standards of privacy rights were applied and no compelling state interest demonstrated.

Androgens and Steroid-Like Substances

This section gathers articles on different hormones other than AAS: DHEA, melatonin, human growth hormone, testosterone, DHT, insulin-like growth factor-1, estrogen, EPO, clenbuterol, salbutamol, and legitimate androgen therapy. There are several articles on the "superhormones," anti-aging hormones, and hormone replacement. DHEA may reverse the decline in strength and muscle mass that comes with aging.

The age of dehydroepiandrosterone, by J. Herbert. LANCET 343:1193-1994, May 13, 1995.
> Commentary on DHEA long thought of as a weak androgen; recommends research trials that take this hormone seriously for anti-aging therapy; references.

Anabolic steroid use in menopause and andropause, by M. G. Di Pasquale. DRUGS IN SPORTS 1:12-13, 1992.
> Therapeutic use of hormone replacement therapy (HRT) in women can provide relief of vasomotor symptoms, prevention of genital atrophy, alleviation of psychogenic manifestations, osteoporosis, coronary artery disease and endometrial hyperplasis/carcinoma; testosterone declines after age 50.

Androgens in men—uses and abuses, by C. J. Bagatell and W. J. Bremner. NEW ENGLAND JOURNAL OF MEDICINE 334(11):707-714, March 14, 1996.
> Reviews the physiology, biologic effects, clinical indications, abuse of androgens, complications and side effects; 91 references. Androgen abuse has become common among athletes and bodybuilders, particularly ones that are difficult to detect, i.e. testosterone.

Attention: aging men, by G. Cowley, et al. NEWSWEEK 128:69-76, 1996.
> General popular audience discussion of hormone replacement therapy for men, including growth hormone, DHEA, testosterone, and melatonin; scrotal patches have been replaced by androderm testosterone patch; DHEA available at health food stores without prescription at much less cost; reports that many men have erection problems after age 50.

Beyond steroids, by S. Veggeberg. NEW SCIENTIST 149:28-31, January 13, 1996.
> Article reports that bodybuilders and weightlifters are using insulin-like growth factor-1 (IGF-1) as an anabolic agent to increase muscle mass, but there are side effects: facial nerve paralysis and edema of the brain. The drug is costly and scarce and intended to treat motor neuron disease and dwarfism.

Blood doping and erythropoietin effects of variation in hemoglobin concentration and other related factors on physical performance, by B. Ekblom. AMERICAN JOURNAL OF SPORTS MEDICINE 24(6):S40-S42, 1996.

Researcher and colleagues studied the effects of external EPO in 24 young men; maximal aerobic and physical performance were enhanced. Results show that it is possible to test for EPO several days after last injection, but did find an increase in BP with EPO administration.

Can this pill really make you younger?, by C. Gorman. TIME 148:66-67, September 23, 1996.

Overview of two books on the wonder drug or dietary supplement, DHEA: Regelson's Super Hormone Promise and DHEA Breakthrough, by Cherniske; DHEA, testosterone and other hormones are promoted as antiaging substances that can slow or reverse aging, but results have been shown on laboratory animals and not humans.

Clenbuterol, a ß-adrenoceptor agonist, increases relative muscle strength in orthopedic patients, by C. A. Maltin, et al. CLINICAL SCIENCE 84:651-654, 1993.

Clenbuterol treatment was associated with more rapid rehabilitation of strength in knee extensor muscles; thus clenbuterol has therapeutic potential for treatment of muscle-wasting conditions. Reviews that salbutamol does not have an ergogenic effect on athletes.

Clenbuterol: muscle growth reported in animals but what effect in humans? PHARMACEUTICAL JOURNAL August 8, 1992, p. 169.

Brief one-page overview of the potential anabolic effect of clenbuterol similar to salbutamol; drug not licensed for human use in UK but available for asthma treatment in Germany, Spain and Italy.

Clenbuterol: a new anabolic drug. DRUGS IN SPORTS 1:3-6, 1992.

This brief article defines and describes the drug used for treatment of asthma which is being increasingly used by athletes for its anabolic properties. Animal studies are reviewed and references listed. Although banned by the IOC it cannot be detected a few days after use.

—, by G. A. Green. SPORTS MEDICINE DIGEST 15:1-3, 1993.

Brief review with research background, clinical applications, adverse effects, drug testing (horse racing first to use), and commentary on athletes quest for magic potion; news item about the British Sports Council transferring clenbuterol into class with AAS because of "anabolic," but controversial because "catabolic"/"anti-catabolic" more correct.

Clinical use of anabolic steroids, by M. G. Di Pasquale. DRUGS IN SPORTS 1:3-4, 1991.

Brief introduction to the legitimate uses of androgens with references.

Dehydroepiandrosterone (DHEA) and aging, by Z. Barrou, et al. ARCHIVES OF GERONTOLOGY AND GERIATRICS 24:233-241, 1997.

This is a very good review of mostly animal but also some human research studies on DHEA and aging and age-related diseases, i.e. cancer, atherosclerosis, osteoporosis, Alzheimer's, and immune response to bacterial or viral infection. Metabolic effects in animals have not been confirmed by substitution trials in humans.

Dehydroepiandrosterone and body fat, by J. N. Clore. OBESITY RESEARCH 3:613S-616S, 1995.
    Studies in man have failed to demonstrate reductions in body fat or increases in metabolic rate; current data do not suggest that DHEA is an effective agent for obesity treatment.

Dehydroepiandrosterone (DHEA): useful or useless as an anti-obesity agent?, by C. D. Berdanier. NUTRITION TODAY 28:34-38, 1993.
    Good overview on DHEA metabolism, obese rat and mice studies, and differences in humans.

Doping at the Olympics: clenbuterol. PHYSICIAN AND SPORTS MEDICINE 20:19-20, 1992.
    Good brief overview with definition, description, desired action for athletes, banned status, etc. which summarizes longer article listed in suggested reading by Di Pasquale.

Drugs sport and the Olympics, by E. Grayson. NEW LAW JOURNAL 142:1171-1172, August 14, 1992.
    This is a brief article about the controversy over clenbuterol because it is a licensed drug in Germany for the treatment of asthma, but not in the UK. Experts disagree about the classification as a stimulant or anabolic agent.

Effect of altered reproductive function and lowered testosterone levels on bond density in male endurance athletes, by K. L. Bennell, et al. BRITISH JOURNAL OF SPORTS MEDICINE 30:205-208, 1996.
    Technical review article which presents the limited literature on the relationship between bone density and testosterone levels in male endurance athletes, but testosterone does not appear to affect bone in males as it does in females.

Effect of recombinant human erythropoietin treatment on blood pressure and some hematological parameters in healthy men, by B. Berglund and B. Ekblom. JOURNAL OF INTERNAL MEDICINE 229:125-130, 1991.
    Expresses concern about increased BP and misuse by athletes to improve performance in endurance events.

Effects of muscle-building exercise on forearm bone mineral content and osteoblast activity in drug-free and anabolic steroids self-administering young men, by C. E. Fiore, et al. BONE AND MINERAL 13:77-83, 1991.
    Found that exercise was major determinant underlying increment of bone density of the radius and that bone loss was slower in menopausal women with higher testosterone.

The effects of supraphysiologic doses of testosterone on muscle size and strength in normal men, by S. Bhasin, et al. NEW ENGLAND JOURNAL OF MEDICINE 335:1-7, July 4, 1996.
    Extra doses of testosterone combined with strength training increase fat-free mass and muscle size and strength in normal men.

Ergogenic aids: clenbuterol, Ma Huang, caffeine, l-carnitine, and growth hormone releasers, by K. E. Friedl, et al. NATIONAL STRENGTH AND CONDITIONING ASSOCIATION JOURNAL 14:35-44, 1992.
    Bodybuilders claim clenbuterol enhances fat metabolism and increases lean muscle mass in humans.

Erythropoietin doping in athletes: possible detection through measurement of fibrinolytic products, by R. Gareau. THROMBOSIS AND HAEMOSTASIS 68:481-482, 1992.

Correspondence from Dr. Gareau reported on laboratory data collected from testing rabbits; potential for detecting the use of rHuEPO for ergogenic aid.

Forever young, by B. Bilger. SCIENCES 35:26-32, 1995.

Reviews the research presented at the DHEA and Aging Conference, sponsored by the NY Academy of Sciences in 1995 (see also Bellino); introduces some of the author-presenters, i.e., Regelson, co-author of Melatonin Miracle; good definitions and explanations of very technical reports and papers.

Growing young, by T. Todd. TEXAS MONTHLY 22(4):46-49, April 1994.

A Texas businessman founded a clinic in Mexico in order to distribute human growth hormone to combat aging , build muscle and reduce fat. The author traveled to the clinic to investigate the claims for hgh treatment. Costs are very high and there are serious side effects.

Growth hormone replacement in healthy older men improves body composition but not functional ability, by M. A. Papadakis, et al. ANNALS OF INTERNAL MEDICINE 124:708-716, 1996.

Healthy older men (70 to 85 years) were given growth hormone to improve functional ability and it was determined that there was modest benefit on body composition, but not significant improvement in muscle strength. Because of side effects and cost, authors do not recommend; exercise achieves greater muscle strength.

Hematological indices of erythropoietin administration in athletes, by I. Casoni, et al. INTERNATIONAL JOURNAL OF SPORTS MEDICINE 14:307-311, 1993.

This study shows the potential method for determining EPO misuse in sports by increases in atypical erythrocytes, but percentages must be established in a wide population.

Hormone craze, by E. DeVita. AMERICAN HEALTH January/February 1996, pp. 70-73.

Reviews the hormones: DHEA, melatonin, growth hormone, insulin-like growth factor, estrogen and testosterone for a popular general audience and mentions some of the current studies being conducted to test the effectiveness of these "anti-aging" products.

Hormone mimics fabled fountain of youth. SCIENCE NEWS 147(25):391, June 24, 1995.

Brief article on the potential of DHEA based on research study in California which treated middle-aged to elderly for a year; showed marked increase in psychological well being; men but NOT women experienced increase in lean muscle mass.

Is dehydroepiandrosterone an antiobesity agent?, by C. D. Berdanier, et al. FASEB JOURNAL 7(5):414-419, 1993.

This reviews the mostly animal studies on DHEA and fatness; some studies report changes in body weight and composition with DHEA. One study showed a decrease in body fat in normal men without a change in body weight. This will have implications for bodybuilders and other athletes should more studies in humans show these benefits.

Is salbutamol ergogenic?: the effects of salbutamol on physical performance in high-performance nonasthmatic athletes, by A. R. Morton, et al. CLINICAL JOURNAL OF SPORT MEDICINE 2:93-97, 1992.
Study examines the effects of the β2 agonist salbutamol on physical performance and lung function of nonasthmatic athletes and concluded that there was no ergogenic effect.

Is this steroid hormone the next miracle fat-loss pill?, by B. Lefavi. MUSCULAR DEVELOPMENT 33:175+, 1996.
Explains what DHEA is, reviews rat studies, warns of side effects, but also reports the potential for health benefits if not for sports and provides references.

Melatonin, by G. Cowley. NEWSWEEK 126:46-49, 1995.
Reviews recent research on melatonin, anti-aging wonder that helps people sleep, boosts the immune system, reduces stress, shows promise as new oral contraceptive, and helps airline workers adjust to different time zones; available cheap in health food stores.

Melatonin efficacy in aviation missions requiring rapid deployment and night operations, by C. A. Comperatore, et al. AVIATION, SPACE, AND ENVIRONMENTAL MEDICINE 67(6):520-524, 1996.
Melatonin appeared to be very effective in maintaining alertness and preventing sleep loss and thus helped military personnel adjust more quickly to a change in time zones. This may have implications for athletes who must travel to international competitions and then be able to perform at their best.

The miracle of melatonin: fact, fancy and future, by D. J. Skene. CHEMISTRY AND INDUSTRY 17:637-640, September 2, 1996.
Author defines melatonin, provides some history of its discovery, briefly explains what is known about the physiology, reviews research results, and discusses the future development; references cited.

Muscling in on clenbuterol. LANCET 340:403, August 15, 1992.
Very good one-page overview with definitions, brief discussion, actions on muscle, review of animal studies, and 13 references.

New age therapy, by L. Jaroff. TIME 147:52, January 23, 1995.
Brief review of the potential benefits of DHEA to halt or reverse the natural decline in strength and muscle mass after age 25; warns that what is sold in health food stores has only very small amounts of DHEA.

New hormone theory, Part II: DHEA update, by M. Colgan. MUSCULAR DEVELOPMENT 33:32+, 1996.
Overview of DHEA's potential and preliminary studies; describes work of Colgan Institute's Hormonal Health Program; references.

The new magic muscle pills, by P. Korn. SELF 15:102+, 1993.
Reports that Barcelona Olympic athletes were sent home who tested positive for clenbuterol, drug used by animal trainers in Europe, but not approved in U.S. Vitamin/mineral supplements also not needed. Chromium, for example, is popular, but await further study as an anabolic or muscle-promoting aid.

Newer uses of growth hormone in adults, by S. L. Kaplan. ADVANCES IN IN-
TERNAL MEDICINE 38:287-302, 1993.
Reviews legitimate medical uses for growth hormone in adults, but it does
not appear to have an advantage for weightlifters in developing muscle
mass.

A phantom killer, by J. Deacon. MACLEAN'S November 27, 1995, p. 58.
Brief report about performance-enhancer EPO, bioengineered form of
erythropoietin and the suspected cause of death of several world-class
cyclists; EPO contributes to cardiovascular abnormalities by thickening
the blood and causing the heart to work harder; still no test to detect the
drug's presence in urine or blood.

Physiological importance of dehydroepiandrosterone, by P. Ebeling and V. A.
Koivisto. LANCET 343:1479-1481, June 11, 1994.
Introduces DHEA and potential positive and negative effects, comparing
benefits for men and women, pre- and post-menopause.

Prostates, pates, and pimples, by J. S. Tenover. ENDOCRINOLOGY AND
METABOLISM CLINICS OF NORTH AMERICA 20:893-909, 1991.
Reviews the known roles for dihydrotestosterone (DHT) in humans and
potential medical uses for steroid 5α-reductase inhibitors. DHT has been
implicated in male pattern baldness, female hirsutism, acne, and enlarged
prostate; extensive references.

Scientific verdict still out on DHEA, by A. Skolnick. JAMA 276:1365-1367,
November 6, 1996.
Warns that although DHEA appears promising as an anti-aging superhormone that can burn fat and build muscle, clinical trials are needed to
verify benefits and that these are for the elderly and long term effects are
unknown; briefly mentions the U.S. Dietary Supplement Health and Education Act of 1994 which allows DHEA to be available without FDA test.

Steroid substitutes, by J. Monroe. CURRENT HEALTH 2 22(8):13-15, April
1996.
Author reports on clenbuterol, chromium, GHB, HGH, and EPO and
warns of health risks; several cases of teen use are briefly described.

Test-driving testosterone, by G. Gutfield. MEN'S HEALTH 9(9):50-51, November
1994.
Testosterone supplementation may be used to build muscle, reduce
belly fat, protect the heart, build stronger bones, but so far the treatment
is for hypogonadism. This article explains and summarizes recent medical
research and suggests that testosterone replacement may be used to
reverse aging.

To build or be built, by R. Laura. SEARCH 25:123-126, May 1994.
This is an essay about growth hormone and genetic engineering, the potential for gene cloning, and the possible impact on bodybuilding.

Use of anabolic steroids in bone disorders, by M. G. Di Pasquale. DRUGS IN
SPORTS 1:5-7, 1991.
Brief article about the use of anabolic steroid therapy to encourage bone
formation; also clearly distinguishes between corticosteroids and anabolic-androgenic steroids; references.

Youth serums: what works, what won't, by B. Lawren. AMERICAN HEALTH
July/August 1997, pp. 52-55+.
Popular magazine article on DHEA, melatonin, human growth hormone,
and life-extending foods.

Training Alternatives

This section gathers articles on nutritional supplements, specifically protein, vitamins, minerals, creatine, energy replacement drinks, ephedrine, plant and herbal products, acetyl l-carnitine, ginseng, and more. A few strength and endurance training alternatives are also discussed.

Acetyl L-carnitine: fat burner, muscle builder or brain booster? This new supplement may do it all, by B. Rowley. JOE WEIDER'S MUSCLE AND FITNESS May 1997, pp. 126-127+.
> Promoted as the "smart drug" to enhance intelligence, acetyl L-carnitine may help keep bodybuilders lean; reviews rat studies and physiology and benefits for older users.

Acute changes in vitamin B_6 status in endurance athletes before and after a marathon, by L. Rokitzki, et al. INTERNATIONAL JOURNAL OF SPORT NUTRITION 4:1554-165, 1994.
> Study to obtain comprehensive vitamin B_6 status of highly trained endurance athletes; technical measurements and values presented.

Anabolic steroids: an alternative [Part 2], by G. Coward. ULTRAFIT 14:55-57+, 1993.
> This author considers some naturally occurring alternatives, but says that animal pituitary gland extracts are useless, sapogenins and sterols are worthless, expensive and dangerous; recommends highly sugared drink ingested within ten minutes of completing intense exercise to increase blood glucose, amino acids, and insulin.

Anabolic steroids substitutes from plant and herbs, by M. G. Di Pasquale. DRUGS IN SPORTS 3:10-15, 1995.
> Warns that some plant and herbal products have misleading advertisements suggesting that they contain natural testosterone or the ability to increase natural testosterone; technical explanation of the production of steroidal hormones; insulin-like growth factor-binding proteins also discussed; references.

Carbohydrates: the complexities of a simple food, by N. Clark. PHYSICIAN AND SPORTS MEDICINE 21(6):49-50+, June 1993.
> Author recommends the best carbohydrates for athletes to enhance their performance and that carbohydrates are better than protein to fuel muscles. She also explains the different requirements for pre- and post-exercise and lists the glycemic index of selected foods.

Chinese caterpillar fungus and world record runners, by D. C. Steinkraus and J. B.
   Whitfield. AMERICAN ENTOMOLOGIST 40:235-238, Winter 1994.
      Coach Ma claimed that the stress-relieving tonic made from caterpillar
      fungus, not drugs, helped his female runners achieve world records; later
      he admitted it was untrue. (See MacLeod, Running Times, February
      1994.)

The Chinese puzzle, by I. MacLeod. RUNNING TIMES February 1994, pp. 28-31.
      Discusses the mysterious training methods of Coach Ma and the sugges-
      tions of drug use; author visited training camp in high altitudes and
      speculates that the Chinese female athletes have always been more suc-
      cessful than men because they have so little opportunity—twelve hours
      of toil in the field for rural peasant women.

Commercially marketed supplements for bodybuilding athletes, by K. K. Grune-
   wald and R. S. Bailey. SPORTS MEDICINE 15(2):90-103, 1993.
      This is an extensive review of twenty different categories of athletic sup-
      plements for bodybuilding. Research data does not support the use of
      these products for ergogenic purposes. Authors are concerned that
      comparisons are often made to anabolic steroids and that athletes might
      see these supplements as safer alternatives. Amino acid mixtures were
      the largest category. This overview is well referenced.

Creatine and its application as an ergogenic aid, by P. L. Greenhaff. INTERNA-
   TIONAL JOURNAL OF SPORT NUTRITION 5:S100-S110, 1995.
      Creatine plays a central role in muscle energy metabolism; this article ex-
      plains the physiology in detail and suggests that it may improve perfor-
      mance in explosive sports and/or high power exercise; extensive refer-
      ences.

Creatine controversy: food or drug?, by B. Lefavi, et al. MUSCULAR DEVELOP-
   MENT 33:172+, 1996.
      Question and answer interview format with several national experts on
      drugs and sports (Voy, Wadler, Yesalis) concerning the potential for crea-
      tine abuse, whether to classify as nutritional supplement or drug, whether
      to ban and test for in competition; DHEA mentioned in comparison and
      doping explained.

Creatine in humans with special reference to creatine supplementation, by P. D.
   Balsom, et al. SPORTS MEDICINE 18:268-280, 1994.
      Provides historical background, physiology, use in sport, treatment and
      adverse effects, and concludes that endurance exercise performance is
      not enhanced, but levels in skeletal muscle can be increased and per-
      formance of high intensity intermittent exercise enhanced following
      creatine supplementation.

Creatine supplementation and exercise performance, by R. J. Maughan. INTER-
   NATIONAL JOURNAL OF SPORT NUTRITION 5:94-101, 1995.
      Creatine supplementation is likely to improve the capacity to maintain
      power output during high intensity exercise, but it may be banned as an
      ergogenic aid.

Diet and athletic performance, by C. K. Probart, et al. MEDICAL CLINICS OF
   NORTH AMERICA 77:757-772, 1993.
      A very thorough and extensive review of dietary supplements, what ap-
      pears to work, from protein to calcium; balanced discussion of research
      results and dietary recommendations for meeting nutritional needs of the
      athlete.

Dietary carbohydrate as an ergogenic aid for prolonged and brief competitions in sport, by J. Walberg-Rankin. INTERNATIONAL JOURNAL OF SPORT NUTRITION 5:S13-S28, 1995.

Depleted carbohydrate is associated with fatigue; recommends high-carbohydrate training diet, carbohydrate beverages during the event, and replacement of carbohydrate stores as soon as possible after the exercise and repeated every hour for five hours. Most likely to help in high power sports when the athlete has lost weight, but certainly for endurance events.

Do athletes need more dietary protein and amino acids?, by P. W. R. Lemon. INTERNATIONAL JOURNAL OF SPORT NUTRITION 5:S39-S61, 1995.

Article suggests that both strength and endurance athletes need more protein than current RDA based on data from sedentary subjects; reviews history, past and present research and recommends more studies on protein/amino acids and exercise.

Don't buy phony "ergogenic aids," by S. Barrett. NUTRITION FORUM 14(3):17+, May/June 1997.

Author warns that extra protein is not needed to build muscle. Protein supplements have been falsely promoted as anabolic without any scientific evidence to support such claims. Sport nutrient products are big business and the FTC has gotten some companies to change advertisements, but the FDA has declined to be involved because the products are not considered drugs.

Effect of strength training and concurrent strength and endurance training on strength, testosterone, and cortisol, by G. Bell, et al. JOURNAL OF STRENGTH AND CONDITIONING 11:57-64, 1997.

Training for both strength and endurance appears to decrease gains for women rowers, but not for men. Researchers measured serum testosterone, urinary cortisol, and strength development.

Effects of creatine supplementation on performance, by B. Ekblom. AMERICAN JOURNAL OF SPORTS MEDICINE 24:S38-S39, 1996.

Brief history and overview of experiments on effects of creatine on exercise; not on IOC doping list but many feel it might be considered doping.

Efficacy of nutritional supplement used by athletes, by S. D. Beltz and P. L. Doering. CLINICAL PHARMACY 12:900-908, 1993.

Reviews findings on efficacy of nutritional supplement and concludes that there is little evidence that they have ergogenic effects in athletes consuming a balanced diet and some have potential harm.

Ephedrine: bodybuilding's hottest new supplement, by J. Feliciano. JOE WEIDER'S MUSCLE AND FITNESS 55(3):110-112+, March 1994.

Provides some historical background on ephedrine, current use as an OTC asthma medication, discusses its potential use for bodybuilding, and the risks . . . also information on mahuang . . . FDA perspective and safety issues. This is a readable and balanced review with some further reading.

Ephedrine's deadly edge, by M. P. Turk. US NEWS AND WORLD REPORT 123(1):79-80, July 7, 1997.

This is a brief article to warn users about the potential dangers of a stimulant extracted from a Chinese herb called mahuang or ephedra. It is considered a dietary supplement and thus not regulated by the FDA, but the FDA has compiled reports of adverse reactions and even death.

Ergogenic aids, by W. Paish. TRACK TECHNIQUE (Winter 1994), pp. 4024-4025.
> Brief explanations, definitions, etc. ATP, creatine, carnitine L, ubiquonone and commentary on energy replacement drinks.

Evaluation of the ergogenic properties of ginseng, by M. S. Bahrke and W. P. Morgan. SPORTS MEDICINE 18:229-248, 1994.
> Explains the varieties of ginseng, effects, doping regulations and concludes that there is only testimonial evidence of ginseng's ergogenic properties.

From ancient Olympia to modern Atlanta: celebration of the Olympic Centennial, by L. E. Grivetti, et al. NUTRITION TODAY 31(6):241-249, 1996.
> Historical background provided as well as summaries of presentations made at a symposium on nutrition and athletic performance; former Olympic athletes are interviewed and their views briefly presented; very extensive references.

How do they do it?, by F. M. Berg. HEALTHY WEIGHT JOURNAL 10:47-48, May/June 1996.
> Brief article about competitive bodybuilding including nutrition and women's issues; very brief information on AAS and eating disorders.

The inside scoop on the hottest workout secrets of top fitness experts, by G. Gutfield. MEN'S HEALTH 10:88+, April 1995.
> Training intermittently is said to burn more fat because less intensity allows muscles to recover and get stronger; weight lifting slowly, visual imagery and more tips.

Low-dose amino acid supplementation: no effects on serum human growth hormone and insulin in male weightlifters, by G. M. Fogelholm, et al. INTERNATIONAL JOURNAL OF SPORT NUTRITION 3:290-297, 1993.
> Authors concluded that low-dose amino acids as supplements do not affect normal daily serum concentration or variation of either hGH or insulin for non AAS-using athletes, namely male weightlifters, despite the belief by athletes that a high protein diet is needed to promote muscle growth.

Nutrition, not steroids, accelerates bodybuilding. BETTER NUTRITION FOR TODAY'S LIVING 55:20+, 1993.
> This article promotes nutritional supplements in order to achieve well-balanced meals and warns against AAS because of side effects. (Refers to an article in the June 1993 issue of Physician and Sports Medicine by Nancy Clark.)

Nutrition supplements: science vs. hype, by T. D. Armsey and G. A. Green. PHYSICIAN AND SPORTS MEDICINE 25(6):77-78+, June 1997.
> Reviews a variety of dietary aids for their ergogenic properties and warns that many do not work, are potentially harmful and costly. Authors conclude that creatine, DHEA, and HMB may have performance-enhancing effects, but no benefits clearly demonstrated for amino acids, L-carnitine, L-tryptophan, or chromium picolinate. DHEA also may effect T/E ratio so that it exceeds the 6:1 limit.

Nutritional ergogenics: help or hype?, by M. H. Williams. JOURNAL OF THE AMERICAN DIETETIC ASSOCIATION 92:1213-1214, 1992.
> Adapted from the presentation, "Ergogenic and Ergolytic Substances," at Nutrition for the Marathon and Other Endurance Sports, April 1992; brief review of ergogenic aids, including vitamins, phosphate salts, etc.

Nutritional supplements for athletes who strength train, by M. Ridgway. PALAESTRA 11(3):23-31, Spring 1995.

Provides interesting historical background on food and nutrition for ancient Greek athletes to modern day protein requirements, amino acid supplements, costs of typical or popular strength training supplements, possible side effects of excess protein and supplements, false labeling and resistance training to build muscle; selected references.

Nutritional supplements: an update for coaches and athletes, by S. J. Massad, et al. PHYSICAL EDUCATOR 53:34-43, 1996.

Discusses protein supplements, steroid alternatives, etc.

Performance-enhancing aids in sport: health consequences and nutritional alternatives, by S. M. Kleiner. JOURNAL OF THE AMERICAN COLLEGE OF NUTRITION 10:163-176, 1991.

Nonsteroid alternatives as well as overview and extensive references—high protein/amino acid supplements—thorough pharmacology and research.

Power plant: can plant sterol ecdysterone help your muscles grow?, by R. Brunner. JOE WEIDER'S MUSCLE AND FITNESS April 1997, pp. 95-96+.

Explains the similarities between plant sterols and anabolic steroids, reviewing Asian and Eastern European studies; recommends diet rich in protein and selected plant sterols to support muscle growth.

Protein supplementation for the scholastic power athlete: a risk and benefits analysis, by F. A. Kulling and B. H. Jacobson. APPLIED RESEARCH IN COACHING AND ATHLETICS ANNUAL (1993), pp. 212-225.

Authors review the importance of protein but do not recommend protein supplements because they can be risky and expensive. They also warn that athletes will be even more tempted to try a more "natural" anabolic product as they are increasingly subjected to drug testing.

A review of nutritional practices and needs of bodybuilders, by J. Walberg-Rankin. JOURNAL OF STRENGTH AND CONDITIONING RESEARCH 9(2):116-124, 1995.

Discusses diet during training and whether supplements are needed; thorough overview with lots of references.

Scuba fitness, by J. Bookspan. SKIN DIVER 41:50-53, 1992.

Brief general overview article on diving and ergogenic aids, i.e. definition of ergogenic, examples, what's good for divers, protein chart, food supplement and enzymes. Warns against using expensive supplements because muscle requirements for protein are very little for growth and most people routinely eat enough in regular diet.

Severe reaction to "natural testosterones": how safe are the ergogenic aids?, by J. M. Pearl. AMERICAN JOURNAL OF EMERGENCY MEDICINE 11:188-189, 1993.

Brief discussion of alternatives to anabolic steroids, similax, illustrated with a case report of an 18-year-old marine who had a severe allergic reaction; hot stuff purchased by the author and literature accompanying the product examined for contents and desired effect, etc.

Testosterone dilemma, by D. R. Sparkman. JOE WEIDER'S MUSCLE AND FIT-
NESS December 1994, pp. 114+.
  Reviews recent findings that fat is necessary for the production of testosterone; recommends maintaining some dietary fat and body fat in order to
  maintain testosterone levels.

The use of nutritional ergogenic aids in sports: is it an ethical issue?, by M. H.
Williams. INTERNATIONAL JOURNAL OF SPORT NUTRITION 4:120-131,
1994.
  Limited research supports the performance enhancing quality of some
  nutrients like creatine when consumed in large amounts . . . i.e. nu-
  traceuticals or nutrients which function as drugs. Williams is editor and
  thus introduces the topic of nutritional supplements, i.e. chromium on
  physical performance which is covered in an earlier issue by another author.

Vitamin/mineral supplement use among athletes: review of the literature, by J.
Sobal and L. F. Marquart. INTERNATIONAL JOURNAL OF SPORT NUTRI-
TION 4:320-334, 1994.
  Thorough review of studies of vitamin/mineral supplement use by athletes, quantified and broken down by gender, sport, etc.; athletes must
  be questioned about excess or megadoses in certain sports, female,
  elite and muscle athletes especially.

What if bodybuilders had never used drugs, by F. C. Hatfield. JOE WEIDER'S
MUSCLE AND FITNESS December 1996, pp. 148+.
  Hatfield's commentary says that neither testing nor education of young
  people will deter drug use; rather an alternative to drug use is needed
  that would provide the same or similar benefits in terms of growth and
  muscular development.

Glossary

AAS
> common abbreviation/acronym for anabolic-androgenic steroids

andropause
> change of life for males, decline in androgen levels in late forties and early fifties

advance notice testing
> athletes know ahead of time when they will be tested either just before competition or shortly thereafter; not considered to be an effective deterrant to steroid use

albuterol (Ventolin or Proventil are trade names)
> long-acting adrenergic bronchodilator, $beta_2$ agonist drug like clenbuterol thought to help with minor strength increases (See also Salbutamol)

aliquot or aliquant
> portion of whole, one of two or more samples of something with same volume and weight as in sample A and B for drug testing, quantity of urine specimen

beta$_2$ agonist (β_2)
> prescription asthma medication which can decrease fat and maintain muscle mass

bromantan
> developed by Russian Institute of Pharmacology in Moscow, may mask testosterone use and thus alter the T/E ratio, may enhance the body's ability to withstand heat stress and boost the immune system, banned by IOC, punishable by four-year suspension

cachexia
> general weight loss and wasting in the course of chronic disease or emotional disturbance

clenbuterol
> asthma treatment prescription medication, disagreement about whether it has anabolic properties or should be classed as a stimulant, banned by the IOC, not licensed for human use in UK or US, but available in Germany, Spain and Italy

creatine
> found in steak or milk and some fish, stored in tissues, also some organs of the body, nutritional supplement thought to enhance high intensity intermittent exercise

cut or cutting
> jargon slang term for muscle definition or body fat burning, also "buffed" for large muscles

DHEA (dehydroepiandrosterone)
> steroid hormone referred to as anti-aging, synthesized from cytosterol found in Mexican yams, may enhance the effects of estrogen in post-menopausal women, may act like an androgen in men and increase lean muscle; adrenal hormone, most abundant steroid hormone in the body

DHT (dihydrotestosterone)
> major androgen which plays a role in acne, male pattern baldness, enlarged prostate and female hirsutism, has anabolic effects; Chinese women tested positive for DHT in 1994 Asian Games, swimmers, weightlifters, etc; also known as stanolone

dragnet testing plans
> drug testing plans which indiscriminately test all students (see also blanket search) purpose to detect and deter student drug use

DSM
> abbreviation or acronym for the Diagnostic and Statistical Manual of Mental Disorders

dumbbell defense
> jargon for the legal strategy wherein psychological and behavioral effects of anabolic steroids are alleged by defendants to have influenced criminal acts; also known as "steroid defense"

dysmorphic
> bad form or disordered shape

ecdysterone
> plant sterol works with the body's natural testosterone to increase muscle protein and growth, can be anabolic in human muscle cells; also known as furostanols

echocardiography
> use of ultrasound to investigate the heart and great vessels and diagnose cardiovascular lesions

endogenous
> produced within the organism

ephedrine
> adrenergic bronchodilator that acts to relax bronchial smooth muscle cells, prescribed in the treatment of asthma and to relieve nasal congest-tion; also contained in over-the-counter dietary supplements (See also mahuang)

EPO

bioengineered hormone erythropoietin used in endurance sports, e.g., cycling, distance running, cross-country skiing, etc.; no test to detect the drug's presence in blood and urine

furosemide

diuretic used for hypertension and edema

gamma hydroxybutyrate (GHB)

causes headaches, nausea, vomiting, diarrhea, seizures, CNS disorders; misinformation that it causes a high, Somatomax PM another name, often in combination with clenbuterol and used to treat narcoleps and may be useful as ergogenic aid

GHRH

abbreviation for growth hormone-releasing hormone

ginseng

roots of several species of Panax, esteemed as of great medicinal value by the Chinese, but not often used in western medicine; used by some Oriental populations as a heart tonic, aphrodisiac and stimulant

glycerol

hyperostotic agent meaning it has the ability to alter osmotic pressure within cells so that the body can hold more fluid; hyperhydration effect to decrease exercising heart rate

glycogen

polysaccharide complex carbohydrate stored in liver and muscles, high-octane fuel

IGF-I

insulin-like growth factor growth enhancer, works best when used with anabolic steroids

individualized suspicion

unconfirmed belief that a certain individual has engaged in illegal activity; nonindividualized directs suspicion towards a group

ischiotibial

anatomical term for connecting the ischium and the tibia, with the ischium being the lower part of the hip bone and posterior and the tibia being the medial and larger two bones of the leg

laurabolin

nandrolone laurate another name, manufactured in Mexico, member of the class of androgens known as 19-nortestosterone derivatives, longer-acting

mahuang

ancient Oriental herb with ephedrine content; used by bodybuilders

melatonin

hormone that promotes sleep, thought to prevent cancer, substance mainly tested on animals, biomarker for age

NCAA
> acronym for the National Collegiate Athletic Association, governing board for college athletics, both public and private colleges and universities; courts have ruled that the NCAA is private and thus not subject to challenge in federal courts or federal constitutional limitations

negative doping or spiking
> administering negative ergogenic or banned substance without the athlete's knowledge so that the person is disqualified

nexus or nexus test
> tie, link or connection between groups, in legal terms, one would have to show a connection between drug use and discipline in order to select for drug testing based on behavior problems; private conduct can be deemed state action if close connection or nexus,for example, the public school and the state

osteopenia
> bone density reduced or reduced bone mass, reduced calcification, sometimes in male athletes

privacy
> legal definitions vary, i.e. protection from exposing one's exterior physical anatomy or from intrusions into one's interior body by way of a urinalysis drug test; the Fourth Amendment of the U.S. Constitution protects against unreasonable searches and seizures

propionibacteria acnes
> P. acnes abbreviated, species of bacteria commonly found in acne pustules, acne bacillus

protropin
> drug approved to treat growth hormone deficiency

pump
> jargon for desired state of muscular congestion in bodybuilding/ weightlifting

reverse anorexia nervosa
> condition in which men who are very large and muscular perceive themselves as being very small; some decline to be seen in public, opposite body-image disorder

salbutamol
> asthma medication which may have an anabolic effect, bronchodilator used for the reversal of symptoms from exercise-induced asthma (See also albuterol)

steroid limp
> damage to the sciatic nerve by injection of anabolic steroids in the buttocks, refers to permanent neuromuscular impairment

steroid psychosis
> severe mental disorder involving changes in personality caused or enhanced by anabolic steroid use

suspicionless searches
      also known as blanket searches, authorized by a legislature and more
      threatening to individual's right to privacy

T/E ratio
      6:1 value exceeding the range normally found in humans, i.e.
      testosterone glucuronide and epitestosterone glucuronide

Author Index

Brief Subject Index